Limited responsibilities

Limited Responsibilities explores the interaction between the criminal justice system and the wider concerns of political and social institutions, including the welfare state, social work and forensic psychiatry.

Using the key concept of 'responsibility', Tamar Pitch critiques the classical theories of Anglo-American and Italian criminologies, examining the allocation of responsibilities to individuals and to society. Looking at the shifting political relationship between criminal justice and the welfare system, Pitch considers the problems which arise in our understandings of responsibility, particularly in relation to the young and the mentally disabled. She also uses the notion of responsibility to explore the contemporary shape of social conflicts, exemplified by women's struggles on sexual violence and the increasing recourse to criminal justice as a symbolic resource by 'victims' of every kind.

Limited Responsibilities will be of interest to lecturers, students and professionals in criminology, social policy and women's studies.

Tamar Pitch is Associate Professor of the Sociology of Law at the University of Camerino, Italy, and a juvenile magistrate. **John Lea** is Head of Criminology at Middlesex University.

SOCIOLOGY OF LAW AND CRIME

Editors: Maureen Cain, *University of the West Indies*
      Carol Smart, *University of Leeds*

This new series presents the latest critical and international scholarship in sociology, legal theory, and criminology. Books in the series will integrate the sociology
of law and the sociology of crime, extending beyond both disciplines to analyse the
distribution of power. Realist, critical, and postmodern approaches will be central
to the series, while the major substantive themes will be gender, class, and race as
they affect and, in turn, are shaped by legal relations. Throughout, the series will
present fresh theoretical interpretations based on the latest empirical research.
Books for early publication in the series deal with such controversial issues as child
custody, criminal and penal policy, and alternative legal theory.

Titles in this series include

Child custody and the politics of gender
Carol Smart and Selma Sevenhuijsen (eds)

Feminism and the power of the law
Carol Smart

Offending women
Anne Worrall

Femininity in dissent
Alison Young

Jurisprudence as ideology
Valerie Kerruish

The mythology of modern law
Peter Fitzpatrick

Interrogating incest
Vikki Bell

Punish and critique
Adrian Howe

Limited responsibilities
Social movements and criminal justice

Tamar Pitch
Translated by John Lea

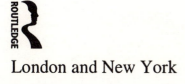

London and New York

This translation first published 1995
by Routledge
11 New Fetter Lane, London EC4P 4EE

Simultaneously published in the USA and Canada
by Routledge
29 West 35th Street, New York, NY 10001

© this translation 1995 John Lea

Responsabilità limitate first published by
Giangiacomo Feltrinelli Editore Milano
© 1990 Tamar Pitch

Typeset in Times by LaserScript, Mitcham, Surrey
Printed and bound in Great Britain by
TJ Press (Padstow) Ltd, Padstow, Cornwall

British Library Cataloguing in Publication Data
A catalogue record for this book is available from the British Library

Library of Congress Cataloging in Publication Data
A catalogue record for this book has been requested

ISBN 0–415–08653–1 (hbk)
ISNB 0–415–08654–X (pbk)

Contents

Preface to the English edition

Since this book came out in Italian, most of what we seemed to have taken for granted has changed, both internationally and in Italy. In a way, when I was twenty I shared the same world as my parents and my grandparents. Though often on different, sometimes antagonistic, fronts, we shared a common language, a similar vision of the world. But that world, or rather the categories we used to interpret (or construct) it, has disappeared. My son will use a different language. But I shan't have to learn it from scratch. Indeed I think that feminism, as a theory and a practice (as theories and practices), has been teaching us for some time already many new languages, and a way to look at the world and our place in it which has anticipated many of the issues which we are confronting today, and which offers more than one way adequately to comprehend and deal with them.

The series of issues I try to deal with in this book refers back to a central one, that of 'responsibility', and the way it is thematised, defined, assumed and attributed in our society (societies). It is not a new issue, but it is one that is today at the centre of public debate, both nationally and internationally. It is the focus of political discussion as well as being a philosophical question and a juridical one. It is the underlying motive of many contemporary conflicts. It may be assumed, and that is what I try to do, as a key to understanding a number of social phenomena. In particular, I use it to understand the interplay between criminal justice institutions and knowledges and welfare institutions and knowledges, and to come to terms with the apparent 'return of the actor' on the social scene. Actors return to the social and political scene, but they are different from those envisaged and constructed by sociologies, philosophies, political theories both of a liberal and socialist type (I do not address postmodern theories directly, but I hope that what I have to say tackles some of the questions they have posed). Feminism's construction of the actor, its sensitivity to responsibility, its introduction into the political lexicon of terms like limit, partiality, positioning, are among its greater contributions, I think, to a language and vision of the world adequate to our times. This book, of course, has much more modest pretensions than what I have so far said seems to imply. I hope that it will at least show one or two new ways to look at criminal justice. New for criminologists, but also for sociologists of law, whose academic ranks I recently joined, after as tortuous an intellectual and academic career as that of many women of my age and background.

This book has been criticised on at least two grounds: because it is more political than analytical, and because it does not provide answers. In a way, I failed twice, I was not scientific enough, I was not political enough. I think both things are true. I wish to think, however, that they do not reflect only my particular way of being 'scientific' and 'political', but that they are also expressions of an approach which privileges questions to answers, flexibility to paradigm construction, open-ended roads to pre-constituted destinations.

This is so true, from a subjective point of view, that I have had problems licensing this translation as John Lea, who, more than a translator, has been a precious interlocutor and wise critic, well knows. Not so much because things go on changing (the things I deal with here do not, fundamentally), but because I have ever more and different questions to pose and because new angles from which I could explore the same issues come continuously to mind. Also many more people have been helping me during these years in reframing my questions than the ones I mentioned in the Italian edition. I wish to thank again Ota De Leonardis, to whose work and intellectual stimulation I shall always be indebted and Maria Luisa Boccia and Ida Dominijanni, without whom I could not be the feminist I am. It is impossible for me to name here all the women from whose work and lives I drew intellectual inspiration, suggestions and support but I wish to re-member Graziella Manfredini who shared with me her thoughts on sexual violence and women's politics about it when already in a hospital bed. Her intellectual sharpness and her capacity for warmth and affection helped me to live after her death.

Franca Faccioli, Giovanna Gallio and Diana Mauri have been precious research colleagues. I want to thank Maria Luisa Boccia, Ota De Leonardis, Ida Dominijanni, Carlo Donolo, Mary Gibson, Marina Graziosi, Luigi Ferrajoli, Raffaella Lamberti, John Lea, Pio Marconi, Guiseppe Mosconi, David Nelken, Massimo Pavarini, Vincenzo Ruggiero and Gabriella Turnaturi for their intelligent and sensitive reviews, comments and presentations of the Italian edition of this book. I grew up academically as a cultural anthropologist. Now that my academic label has changed to that of sociologist of law, I wish to thank Tullio Seppilli for orienting me towards the study of deviance and social control, and all my friends at the Istituto di Antropologia Culturale dell'Universita di Perugia for providing me with a stimulating environment where I could freely address these issues, when so many still thought they were outside the domain of cultural anthropology; Alessandro Baratta and the editorial boards of *La Questione Criminale* and *Dei Delitti e delle Pene* for providing me with the chance of pursuing these studies within the framework of criminology and sociology of law; Luigi Ferrajoli for opening up to me new avenues into the study of law and new ways for me to look at the politics of law.

My intellectual debt to Stanley Cohen will be clear to whoever reads this book. I met Stan Cohen in the 1970s through the European Group for the Study of Deviance and Social Control. To this group I owe the chance of coming into contact with students of many countries and of establishing fruitful intellectual relationships with them. I would not have attempted to publish this book in English without the encouragement and help of Maureen Cain and Carol Smart. As I already mentioned, John Lea's work on this book has gone much beyond that of translation. He has been interpreter, critic, discussant and helped me to try to reframe questions having in mind an English-speaking audience. If I have failed, it is through no fault of his. Finally I wish to thank Nicola Gallerano, companion and father of my son. As a student of contemporary history, he offered a special angle from which to look at the issues I deal with here, plus a great deal of help in the art of controlling a word processor.

This book is dedicated to my parents, Mirella Sadun and Eric Pitch, and to my son David who was not yet born when it was first written.

Rome, 12 July, 1993

Preface to the Italian edition

A central place in this book is occupied by the criminal justice system. But this is not a book about the criminal justice system as such. It does not define it or discuss its functions – manifest or latent. Rather the criminal justice system is the place where or around which many of the processes described here take place. But it is not the object of the book even if I maintain and hope that by means of these processes people acquire different perspectives from which to look at criminal justice. In this sense criminal justice is the object of the book but not directly. It is rather an arena of conflict or a symbolic resource of collective actors, an articulation of the politics of social control.

Studies of the criminal justice system viewed as articulations of social control are in Italy still relatively few in number. That has to do with a particular interpretation of this category in Italian intellectual culture, an interpretation which has made difficult the exploration of the connections between different systems which can be viewed as components of the structure of social control. Thus a primary theoretical and methodological focus of the book consists in analysing the category of social control and the uses for which it has been adapted, reviewing its history and offering an interpretation of it which adequately accommodates also studies of the criminal justice system. The rich tradition of foreign studies, above all Anglo-Saxon, has to be gone over again critically to argue for the necessity of a reading of the system of criminal justice from the standpoint of interaction with other systems of social control. The result is an analysis of the present politics of social control different from that prevailing both in Italy and elsewhere, and there follows a methodological and theoretical polemic with the dominant currents in critical sociology on these issues, a polemic which argues for the abandonment of those fundamentalist perspectives which renounce the link between theory and the search for effective political solutions.

It is crucial in the analysis of the criminal justice system, as with that of other agencies of social control, to grasp the dynamic and processual aspects of control and to understand its effects as the product, not only of interaction, through both negotiation and conflict, between the agencies, but also between those agencies and their users. This throws light on a hitherto neglected aspect, namely, criminal justice as a point of inter-section, a symbolic resource and observation post for questions, exigencies, conflicts, not only for the agencies themselves but also for social actors and movements. The great theme which emerges from this focus is that of *responsibility*, a theme currently at the centre of sociological, philosophical, juridical and political debates.

I analyse the connection between the attribution and assumption of responsibility in the context of the crisis of the welfare state or the culture of welfare, both in relation to models of the institutional administration of social problems, the culture of the professionals, and in relation to the participants in everyday conflicts. On the one hand I am concerned with two cases which symbolise the crisis in the relationship between criminal justice and the structure of social and psychological welfare. The situations of mentally ill offenders and of juvenile offenders both serve to highlight issues relating to the attribution and assumption of responsibility and the contrast between civil and social rights.

On the other hand the theme of responsibility also emerges in the relations between care and autonomy expressed in the demands which collective actors make on the criminal justice system. The emergence of demands for the criminalisation of social problems exhibits an oscillation between demands for care and the requirements of autonomy, these demands find a provisional and contradictory landing place in the con-frontations of a de-subjectivising and de-responsibilising culture. But the case which I examine most deeply is the campaign by sections of the women's movement in Italy for a new law on sexual violence, which opens up further considerations which anchor the problematic of responsibility and, equally widely discussed, of the relations between (or the politics of) equality and the (politics of) difference. These relations embrace in reality, without becoming recognised in such terms, all the interactions between the criminal justice system and institutions of welfare, care and protection which appear in a new light when they are seen from the standpoint of demands which women put on the criminal justice system.

Around the questions of equality and responsibility and difference finally converge (miraculously it seems to me, but in reality, as I intend to argue, it is not at all an accident) the diverse paths and the diverse bits of my intellectual and political biography, and various focuses of my research activities. This is a provisional reflection on years of work and political experience (with women principally) often on questions which from time to time I saw as separate and different one from the other. And naturally they are. But it is what unifies them that I am concerned with and which I have tried to reconstruct here.

I have had the help of many people, above all those with whom I have worked over the last ten years in various research projects, in the editorial work of the reviews *La Questione Criminale* and *Dei Delitti e delle Pene*, in the arena of feminist politics. Together with them I would like to thank those who have read and commented on one or other chapters of this book, Maria Luisa Boccia, Gaetano de Leo, Ota De Leonardis, Nicola Gallerano. Their criticisms and suggestions were vital to me. It goes without saying that the responsibility for errors and omissions is mine alone.

Rome, September, 1989

Series editors' preface

This is the last book in our limited series on the Sociology of Law and Crime. It is a fitting final work, because it quite explicitly attempts to achieve that objective which was the *raison d'être* of the series as we conceived it: a shift in focus and a transformation of sociological thinking in relation to crime and law resulting from an application and acceptance of feminist work.

Tamar Pitch writes from the perspective of someone actively and above all reflexively engaged in feminist struggle. But this is not a book only about women. Indeed, when women do appear they are such active political and theoretical participants that we forget their gender: there must be a lesson here! Pitch's aim is to use the experience of the struggles which she knows so well, the gains and the losses in relation to rape, to abortion, to learn lessons about law and about progressive political practice on behalf of all oppressed people. In this way the searchlight of feminist experience is turned on critical criminology in general.

In order to attempt this ambitious project Pitch used the key concept of 'responsibility'. This concept is the scalpel with which she dissects the classical theories of Anglo-American liberal and critical criminologies as well as the very different Italian tradition, more polarised politically until the English language texts made their mark.

Responsibilities are allocated to individuals and society, they can also be claimed or accepted politically. The ideological interplay of these processes of displacement and reclamation exposes the strategies of criminologists and administrators alike.

Pitch's own research has been on child offenders ('so-called juvenile delinquents') and on the rights of the mentally ill, while her practice-related work has been concerned with more specifically female issues. All these oppressed groups use, need, collude with, and are constrained by welfare services, and this complex interrelationship provides the second theme of this work. Again the concept of the allocation of responsibility is used as the axis against which theoretical distinctions and political evaluations are made. The particular struggles, which like all struggles must be local, are given universal significance by the opportunities for conceptual elaboration – and strategic insights – which they provide.

The heart of the argument for us – although we do not know if the author would agree – lies in chapter 7, where the consequences of a theoretical and ideological shift from a concept of oppression to a concept of victimisation are explored. This connects directly with those forms of radical victimology which have been so much debated in the pages of critical criminological journals in recent years, and also demonstrates, for women and all oppressed groups, the dangers of accepting the substitution of pity for politics.

This is an analysis infused – as we intended all the books in this series to be – with passion and commitment. It is the more effective because these are expressed with restraint, almost disguised, and a rare intellectual refinement. It is therefore a fitting work with which to conclude this series of nine books. With the contributions of Professor Pitch and our other eight authors we have clearly come very close to achieving our goals of not just 'integrating' feminist and other critical criminologies and sociologies of law, but also of re-theorising the core of these disciplines in the light of feminist knowledges. So we have begun the work of producing a truly engendered mainstream, however broad and diverse its currents and tributaries may continue to be.

Maureen Cain
Carol Smart
October, 1993

Acknowledgements

Some the material of this book has appeared either in its present form or in earlier versions elsewhere. Some of the issues developed in chapter 1 were anticipated in my essay 'Che cos'e il controllo sociale' in O. De Leonardis, G. Gallio, D. Mauri, T. Pitch (eds.) 1988, *Curare e Punire* (Milano, Unicopoli). An earlier shorter version of chapter 3 appeared in *Inchiesta* nos. 79–80 1988. Chapter 4 previously appeared in a different form in F. Faccioli, T. Pitch (eds.) 1988, *Senza Patente* (Milano, Franco Angeli). Chapter 6 previously appeared as 'La sessualità, le norme, lo stato' in *Memoria* No. 17, 1986.

1 Processes and products of social control

The use and abuse of a concept

The concept of social control has a long and controversial history not only within sociology, whose development it accurately mirrors, but also in political science, anthropology and social psychology. It is not my intention to retrace this history. Rather, in a book whose central focus of attention is the criminal justice system, I would like to single out, through an analysis of some of the applications of the concept, the ways in which it can be used to situate the criminal justice system itself and to understand aspects of it which have hitherto been rather hidden in the Italian literature.

Social control is a concept imported from the English speaking world and its current usage, both in everyday speech and in the social sciences, is relatively recent in Italy. I will deal in the next chapter with what I consider to be the specifically Italian aspects of the study of crime and the criminal justice system. Italian sociology in general appears to have touched only peripherally on questions which in other intellectual traditions come under the heading of social control. Rather, such questions have been constructed in a different way and therefore discussed under different headings. This has to do with the interplay between a specific cultural tradition and the particular development of questions which in other cultures are interpreted through the category of social control.

The term 'social control' derives from a tradition of philosophy and political theory whose roots lie within the framework of a complex decentralised democracy with an ethnic and cultural diversity. In such a context the term has performed differing and even contradictory tasks. It has formed the basis both of an account of the various forms of self regulation of the social system, and of the dynamics of social integration in a multi-ethnic society. Obviously I am referring here to the United States where the category of social control was not only coined for the first time (by E.A. Ross), at least as a central concept in sociology, but was adopted within the most diverse theoretical models, functioning as a description of, and as a response to, political, social and cultural questions which changed both over time and between particular fields of study.

The concept of social control theorises the problem of social order in fundamentally anti-Hobbesian terms. As the central issue in European social science for a century, the question of order was posed in Europe in terms of a relationship between the individual and society which is basically conflictual and in which human nature is by no means entirely socially determined. There is thus a double dualism, detectable in different ways both in Durkheim and in Freud, which tends to become obscured in the reconceptualising of the problem of social order as that of social control. It is the consequent fading of this dualism which helps to explain the continual transition, in the American social science tradition, from the macro to the micro levels of social control: from the regulation of the social system to the induction of the individual into social conformity. It is this fading, finally, which explains the semantic extension and the multiple uses of the interface of social control: the concept of deviance.

The concept of social control is, as I have noted, of relatively recent importation into Italian intellectual culture. It is being utilised today with a suspect abundance: suspect in my opinion because it betrays little awareness of the debates of which social control was and is the subject. Until not long ago most of the questions now being formulated in terms of social control were theorised in other ways: as questions having to do with power, domination and hegemony. To what new demands and/or changes in theoretical standpoint does the deployment of the concept of social control correspond?

REGULATION, CONFORMITY, CONSENSUS, COERCION

In a famous article Morris Janowitz (1975) spoke out in defence of a 'high' connotation which, in his words, the concept of social control possessed in the classical sociological tradition. The macro sociological origins of the term had, argued Janowitz, become successively banalised in order to identify the micro, or rather the psycho-social, processes involved in the induction of individuals into conformity with social norms. This supposed banalisation in reality is already implicit in the very transformation of the problem of social order into that of social control. It is therefore not so much a question of trivialisation as of privileging one of the several possible lines of enquiry implied in that transformation. Of course the choice of, or rather the exclusive emphasis on, the micro processes of social control identifies particular theoretical orientations different from those which would follow from an emphasis on the so called 'macro' side of the issue.

In a suggestive analysis Melossi (1983) situates the emergence of the problematic of 'social control' in two interrelated transitions: an historical transition from the late feudal absolutist and the classical nineteenth century liberal states to that of modern complex democracy, and a theoretical transition from the science of politics and law to social science. When social order is seen as a natural result of the free interplay of economic forces in which the role of the state is limited to that of guarantor – a model, as Melossi points out, both normative in the form of the ideology of 'laisser faire', and interventionist in allocating to political organisation the task of removing all resistance to capitalist development – the state itself is perceived only as law, that is, as that which guarantees juridically the 'natural rights' of the bourgeois citizen. But when the problem is posed of a law which not only reflects, but also actively intervenes in, the functioning of the market, such a system of law cannot be understood simply as the expression of civil society, but refers directly to 'the state' as an – ethically superior – institutional entity.

The spread of democracy during the later 19th and 20th centuries through the enlargement of political citizenship and the recognition and institutionalisation of social conflict dissolved the unity of the ethical state and displaced the problem of social order onto new terrains and new bodies of knowledge. Such circumstances formed the background to the development of European sociology. But it was especially the North American social sciences which confronted these issues from the standpoint of social control. This, according to Melossi, was due to the anti-statist tradition of American political theory and to a cultural environment marked by pragmatism and by its attention to the active and processual aspects of human experience. The problem of social order, or how ethical cohesion and social organisation arise in a non coercive way, is transformed into the problem of social control.

I would like to emphasise three aspects of this transformation. First, and this is the aspect underlined by Melossi, is the substitution in the American sociological tradition of social control for the state, by contrast with the European tradition in which the latter retains its centrality. One of the most interesting consequences of this substitution seems to me to be that of decentralisation. The sites of the production of social order multiply, diffuse and disperse themselves outside of any hierarchy. This poses nevertheless a fundamental problem: that of explaining, identifying or reinforcing the coherence between the various forms of social control in the absence of a central, hierarchically co-ordinated process.

The second aspect relates to the attenuation, in the concept of social control, of the conflict between individual and society, human nature and culture. The theory of symbolic interactionism, which draws its foundations from the social psychology of G.H. Mead (1966), in its turn closely linked to pragmatist philosophy, conceives the personality as the product of communicative inter-action and therefore as entirely social. This does not signify a disappearance of the tension between individual and society, rather the nature of that tension changes in such a way as to no longer presuppose a fundamental irreducibility of one to the other. Symbolic interactionism is a theoretical and methodo-logical current which runs through the entire American sociological tradition. In various interpretations and deployments it inspired the Chicago School (and, in conjunction with other theoretical currents of European origin, such as phenomenology, later tendencies deriving from the Chicago School – for example, ethnomethodology and labelling theory) just as it inspired structural functionalism.

The third aspect concerns the semantics of order and control. To re-theorise the problem of social order as a problem of social control implies a displacement of emphasis from mechanisms of government 'of' actions whose social nature is prior to and independent of such regulation, to processes of intervention 'in' events which only derive their social nature as a result of such intervention. This shift entails both a subjectivisation and a depoliticisation of the process of control. It becomes subjective in the sense that control refers back to interventions, by something or someone, oriented to, or interpretable by reference to, goals and values. It is de-politicised because these interventions are generalised and dispersed and their analysis starts from the question of 'how do they function?' rather than to that of 'what type of order do they produce?'[1]

In Europe, as in the United States, it is the non-coercive aspects of the production of social order which are of interest. But where, as in Europe, the state remains the central question, these aspects can only be understood as founded on domination. When, on the other hand, social control is substituted for the State, this foundation tends to disappear. Again, two general consequences of these different approaches can be identified. The first has to do with the identification of the object of analysis itself. Much of what in the American sociological tradition is analysed through the category of social control, in the European tradition is the subject matter of political science, political sociology and the sociology of organisation. In other words, traditional European reflection on the question of order has confronted the problems of social integration as institutional and political problems rather than as problems of conformity and deviance.

The second consequence is that social control, in the dominant American tradition, indicates a generative – as opposed to repressive – process. Various theoretical schools see social control as productive of consciousness, personality, identity, organisation and as implying complex processes of interaction.

Social control involves therefore not only the macro processes of social organisation and social integration, but also the micro processes which induce individual conformity or which, to put it another way, produce consensus or shared meanings as an end result. The emphasis on the processual and productive aspects of social control is accentuated in those types of analysis which focus on the dynamics of the production of meaning. It is less evident in those in which the sharing of meaning – consensus – is explicitly taken as a starting point. Among the first are those interpretative models derived from the classical version of symbolic interactionism, rooted in the social psychology of G.H. Mead, while among the second, structural functionalism as developed both by Merton and Parsons is pre-eminent.

In the social psychology of Mead the self is formed and transformed by the individual subject in a process of self reflection on the ways in which she imagines others to perceive her. The relation with others is therefore constitutive of the self to the extent to which the latter, through a process of interpretation, adopts attitudes of significant others in specific situations. The fundamental process at work here is that of communication mediated by symbols and primarily by language. The emphasis is on the self-reflective aspect of interaction. This process of self reflection leaves room for the interpretation of what makes communication possible: the sharing of symbols and meanings. This process of interpretation is the dynamic aspect of interaction. The sharing of meanings – consensus – can then be analysed not as a presupposition but as a product of continuous negotiations. Social control, in this perspective, becomes a property of any interaction. It is *self*-control, or rather the process of internalisation by the self of the attitudes of others through confrontation with, and adjustments to, the latter. Social control proceeds from self reflection on the effects of interaction.[2]

It is this negotiated character of norms which disappears in structural functionalism. The Parsons of *The Social System* (Parsons 1965) resolves the Hobbesian problem of order in radically anti-Hobbesian terms. If order, which is here taken to mean consensus, is what the theory has to explain, it does so only by taking consensus itself as its presupposition. Consensus – that is, collective orientation through shared values – is a functional prerequisite of the general system of action. It is not therefore really the process of the construction of consensus that the theory sets out to analyse, but rather how such consensus maintains and reproduces itself. The interpenetration of the personality and cultural systems takes place through the complete internalisation of values by the personality. Such values then constitute the motivational structure of the personality. This is, it could be said, a circular solution. It lacks the self-reflexive dynamic and the anchoring in a specific situation characteristic of interactionist psychology. It is the entirely social self which is in evidence here (see Giddens 1979 among others) such that, as has been noted, one cannot speak of action in Parsons so much as of behaviour or rather conduct entirely determined by normative role expectations. The processes of socialisation are at one and the same time processes of social control. The prototypical mechanism of 'secondary' social control, or response to deviance, is, for Parsons, psychotherapy as the model of a relationship which attempts to reconstruct the missing motivational links to values through a technique which makes deliberate use of those attitudes of detachment and sustained support typical of a process of successful socialisation.[3]

In the American sociological tradition therefore, the concept of social control describes a domain[4] of processes and institutions in which the criminal justice system, indeed law itself, occupy a peripheral and residual place.[5] They are those processes and institutions of 'expert' intervention which, by taking charge of aspects of social behaviour defined as problematic, both reinforce and substitute for the agencies of primary socialisation. Their mode of operation is a repetition of the forms of socialisation themselves. Very early on (see Ross 1922, and the subsequent development of the Chicago School), and at the same time as these institutions developed and multiplied, the question of social order is established as that of the production of motivations for action rather than the censuring and sanctioning of behaviour.[6]

By contrast, the adoption of the concept of social control by a theoretical perspective characterised by some form of dualism has different results. Here control is interpreted as either a process of prohibition and interdiction or as the production of 'inauthentic' motivations, or both. In all three cases it is assumed that the source of control is exogenous, either to the social system as such, in the form of 'nature', of environment to the social system, or else as that area of the social which is dominated and colonised. The effect is either to relocate the diffusion of social control as a process which is extraneous or overdetermined with respect to the individual actor or to denote by control only those exogenous processes which intervene to alter supposedly 'self-governing' forms of regulation which are then assumed to be expressive of the true needs and interests of the actors involved. In this theoretical scenario the criminal justice system, even more than law, is central.[7] By starting from the centrality of the criminal justice system and from the logic of censure, sanction and repression which are imputed to it, other processes of social control, located elsewhere and operating with different dynamics, are understood as auxiliary processes which function to produce inauthentic motivations or which censure behaviour by other means.[8]

These two treatments of social control have to do more with the different political cultures from which they emanate than with any significant difference in the importance of punitive institutions and the dynamics of power in American and European societies, even though of course these cultures themselves arise from different experiences of conflict and its management. It is sufficient to think of Keynesianism and the 'New Deal' on the one hand and of European fascism on the other. Today however, these two interpretations coexist in countries with similar political configurations and comparable proliferations of specialist institutions oriented to intervention in, and assumption of responsibility for, social problems. Indeed, the second – European – understanding of social control achieved considerable popularity in the United States during the 1960s and 1970s. What took place in fact during this period was on the one hand the adoption of the concept of social control in European sociological and political debates, and on the other the penetration of dualistic models into the North American sociological environment. It is precisely this process of interpenetration of the two traditions which has been conducive to an elaboration of social control as concerned with processes and institutions which are simultaneously totalizing and oppressive.

THE MERITS AND DEMERITS OF DUALISM: TOWARDS A DEFINITION

For a long time the two interpretations of social control have been representative, the first of a consensual and the second of a conflict-oriented theory of social dynamics. The literature on this is enormous (see the bibliography in Pitch 1982) and refers to a context of debate, now quite dated, typical of the early 1970s.

The penetration of at least the terminology of social control and deviance into Italian sociology – which has always had a strongly dualistic theoretical horizon – is due, it seems to me, to two main factors. On one side the explosion, since the late 1960s, of a wide spectrum of social conflicts involving previously unknown social actors and taking place very much outside traditional areas of struggle. In such conflicts the term 'deviance' lent itself, and was often utilised by the protagonists themselves, to describe and integrate a diversity of conflicts into a common frame of reference: this frame of reference was the sharing of a common antagonistic subjectivity or of a situation of oppression to which the working class gave meaning and practical expression. 'Social control' thus served to identify a range of processes and institutions much more extensive than that invoked by the category of 'repression'. The attribution of social control became a weapon for actors involved in conflict who 'discovered' hitherto unrevealed modes and sites of oppression, or denounced as oppressive social conditions and situations hitherto considered normal.

The second reason for the popularity of the terminology of social control is that it has enabled the coexistence of custodial institutions such as prisons, mental hospitals etc. and more decentralised forms of organisation and treatment oriented approaches to social problems, to be grasped as different aspects of a unified strategy. However, although this resulted in a critical and vigilant attitude towards decentralisation, it often led those concerned primarily with the criminal justice system to accord the latter a central and fundamental role in the shaping of the new processes.

Dualistic paradigms of social control grasp the standpoints of the actors of social conflicts but pretend to found them in some outside place: in nature, 'real' needs, 'unrepressed' desires, contradictions of the system etc., from which the 'true' meaning of these standpoints can be derived. Dualist paradigms make possible the identification of 'points of resistance', which allows the attribution of rationality to conflicts and the taking into account of the dynamics of power. But conflict and interaction remain abstract dynamics and the two poles of the dichotomy – actors and their 'real' needs on the one hand, the system of social control on the other – remain mutually non-reducible, thereby consigning both to an a priori status which itself negates a reading in terms of conflict and interaction. The end result is either a voluntarism of eternal conflict of actors versus system, or a determinism of total colonisation of the actors by the system.

It is not necessary however to found the actor's standpoint within an external and causal relationship to social conflict and interaction. The point of view of the actor is, on the contrary, itself a product of the process of interaction and its claims to rationality can only be validated in that context. The 'externality' of social control to the actor has to be understood as shifting. It is not simply a process of resistance to imposition but is rather constructed within the dynamic of conflict and interaction with forces perceived both as producing conformity and as imposing constraint. Such interaction leads in its turn to the production of new norms, new boundaries and definitions of 'normality'.

In a model of this type the concept of social control is enriched rather than impoverished by its ambiguity. By making it possible to understand different processes – of socialisation and coercion – in terms of the production of motivations, it allows us to see how different spheres of social life and different institutional competencies interrelate and overlap. It also permits us to refer at the same time to a particular social organisation and to the experience and interpretation of that organisation.

This conception of social control has evolved in the context of the interventionist welfare state. The concept fulfils two interconnected functions. First, it serves to identify those processes which simultaneously produce both 'consensus' and 'coercion', or which are one or the other – depending on the standpoint from which they are analysed. Secondly, it exhibits the inter-connections between processes which operate in different ways with different objectives: intervention on 'neglect' and poverty, the politics of health care, psychiatry, and the politics of crime and public order.

To define such processes as ones of social control is a choice: they can also be analysed in other terms. Social control does not identify a specific object so much as it forms a conceptual starting point. The study of which processes are at various times identified as social control is, on the other hand, illuminating for the understanding of the transformation and dis-placement of social conflicts. What is identified as 'control' – or its effects – depends in large measure on the emergence of actors who, reclaiming an autonomous political and social subjectivity, denounce as forms of control, or obstacles to the attainment of such subjectivity, spheres of activity hitherto enacted and lived as neutral.

In this book I am concerned with some of the social groups and institutions which interact with the criminal justice system as part of the process of articulation of ideas and strategies based on definitions of 'good' and 'normal'.

I would argue that anyone who in the present period seeks to understand the production of social control must take into account at least three areas, or types of processes. Firstly, those relating directly to law and the criminal justice system[9] and also to psychiatry and psychiatric institutions (areas which have hitherto, as we shall see, been the predominant focus in the Italian literature on this theme). Secondly, those imputed to agencies involved in the distribution of services and resources (such as health care, income support), to the extent to which such operations base themselves on and contribute to the articulation of notions of 'good' and 'normal'. Thirdly, those relating to the activities of social groups and movements as producers of notions of 'good' and 'normal', in their confrontation with such institutions.[10]

THE CRIMINAL JUSTICE SYSTEM AND OTHER SYSTEMS OF SOCIAL CONTROL: A RECENT DEBATE

The principal interlocutors of the debate on the nature, orientation and signi-ficance of the policies of contemporary social control are however still the sociologists and criminologists who see social control as the institutions and processes defining and administering deviance (Cohen 1985). This definition, as I have argued elsewhere (Pitch 1988), is tautological and furthermore assumes a centrality of crime and criminal justice which gives an exaggerated coherence and unidirectionality to the sources and production of social control. It is useful nevertheless to go over this debate once again because of its importance in laying down the present terrain of discussion and research.

At the centre of the debate is the interpretation of changes which took place during the 1960s and 1970s. During these years, albeit in different ways and at different rates in various countries, there evolved a dominant discourse of and about social control apparently united in its focus on decriminalisation, deinstitutionalisation, decentralisation and territorial- isation. Nevertheless the polemics and discourses around social control were, in fact, a reflection of diverse and contradictory processes occurring in different national situations.

In the United States and in Great Britain the 'new discourse' of social control (Cohen 1985) emerged in a context of a developed welfare state and took the form of a critique of the oppressive and disciplinary results of welfare. It nevertheless initially took for granted a horizon of steady incremental increases in public spending. It is a discourse characterised by tolerance and permissiveness (for Great Britain see NDC 1980) exem- plified by support for alternatives to custody, decriminalisation of 'crimes without victims', and psychiatric deinstitutionalisation, alongside exhor- tations to the tolerance of 'diversity' and non-conformist life styles. This entailed a defence of individual rights against the paternalistic and 'thera- peutic' welfare state and took the form of a reorientation of the politics of welfare towards client participation, decentralisation and community control (see Nelken 1985, Scull 1982). These latter were seen as the basis for a non-therapeutic re-socialisation, freed from disciplinary connotations and answering to needs defined by clients. This type of welfare policy proposal found a reflection in sociology in the work of the labelling theorists. As far as the area of criminal justice was concerned, the issues were depenalisation and decarceration (Scull 1977), put into practice parti- cularly in the area of 'juvenile delinquency' through elaborate diversion schemes making maximum use of probation and community service.[11]

This epoch of reforms came, nevertheless, to be judged with extreme severity. From the 'left' their effects were denounced as conducive to a diffusion of control and surveillance into new areas and populations hitherto excluded. Decentralisation and community involvement were seen as the extension of a 'soft' control which had not replaced segregation and custody so much as added to them with the effect of 'spreading the net' of bureaucratic institutional interventions, (see Cohen 1988)[12] and further eroding the areas both of legitimate political conflict and debate and of private and individual spaces.

This pessimistic reading, evident in much of the Anglo-Saxon literature, is associated with the introduction of a theoretical model derived from Marxism into the conventional paradigms of the sociology of social con- trol. Based on a traditional typology of conflict, such an approach is incapable of grasping new modalities of social control which are now increasingly important. Forms of control progressively less repressive and more technical, administrative and welfare oriented are seen as inexorably invading every aspect of social life, meeting little resistance. The dimension of conflict is grasped only up to the point at which social policies are translated into law, the effects of which are then interpreted as substantial successes of 'power'. What this model is unable to grasp, a point to which we will refer frequently later, is the transformation produced by the spread of a culture of welfare: in particular the continual and irreversible lowering of the threshold of legitimate access to a social and political response to issues and interests hitherto considered as 'natural'.

A progressive de-naturalisation has thus occurred, a symptom of which is, among other things, a marked increase in the symbolic use of criminal justice with regard to areas such as the administrative and the economic, where it functions as a legitimation of new interests. This will be the focus of chapter 3.

From the political 'right' on the other hand, welfare and the reforms inspired by it were denounced as useless, inefficient and costly. In the United States the politics of neo-liberalism advocated a return to a strict retributivism in terms of social defence. Law and order campaigns, differently motivated in different countries (in Italy, terrorism, drugs and organised crime, in Great Britain, street crime. See Hall *et al.* 1978 and then the riots of the black ghettos, see Lea and Young 1984) rejected both the 'new' strategies of re-socialisation and the 'old' ones of re-education and rehabilitation. This will be discussed in chapter 2.

A particularly suggestive characterisation of the present scenario is provided by the metaphor of 'bifurcation' through which social control policies are seen as increasingly moving in two separate directions. On one side there is the development of explicitly repressive and segregated custodial regimes, symbolised by a prison purged of any re-educative illusions and oriented directly to the incapacitation of a residual hard core of untreatable offenders. Differentiation as the new model of prison management is part of this logic.[13] The other side of the coin would appear to be the spread of a 'soft' control, informed by therapeutic and treatment perspectives. Decentralised and community based, it is oriented towards 'the rest': petty offenders, juvenile delinquents construed as a population capable of being reclaimed and re-socialised through education, rehabilitation and re-socialisation (see Pavarini 1986).

SOCIAL DANGEROUSNESS: A BOUNDARY QUESTION

In the literature on the criminal justice system, the renewed fortunes of the category of 'social dangerousness' is interpreted as the outcome of the crisis of the strategy of penal reform. It is certainly true that social dangerousness as a concept is enjoying new and increasing favour. It now functions as a legitimation for incapacitation, as the criterion of classification within the prison itself and between custodial strategies as such and the policies of 'soft' control. Social dangerousness resurfaces as the counter to the 'rehabilitation' model. It can therefore function both as a key to an understanding of the present policies of control and as a standard from which to judge the prevalent liberal and 'left' theories. As the illegitimate offspring of the crisis of welfare policies, this renewed idea of dangerousness has lost the biological positivist connotations which it originally carried and has acquired connotations which facilitate the extension of its use (De Leonardis 1988). It functions as a residual category: all that which is not amenable to treatment or rehabilitation is therefore dangerous.

Nevertheless the metaphor of bifurcation (prevalent in 'left' interpretations of social control policies), by starting from the standpoint of the criminal justice system, only grasps those aspects of contemporary social dangerousness which immediately legitimise it. It is deployed, in other words, to describe and manage phenomena portrayed as irredeemably immune to any form of rehabilitation or soft control: the terrorist, the mafiosi and those by definition non-rehabilitable by virtue of being consciously in conflict with the rules of the social pact. From this starting point the literature proceeds to interpret the extension of the category of social dangerousness to include 'violent' and 'really serious offenders' (Bottoms 1977) as a way of minimising the costs – economic and symbolic – of the incarceration model. This would enable the latter to re-legitimise itself as the strategy of last resort to cope with social conflicts reduced to, or represented by, 'groups divided into the mad and the bad' (Bottoms 1977 p. 87), while measures of decarceration, depenalisation, supervision in the community, would be extended to all those categories of offenders for whom situational theories still retain some plausibility.

But this reading in terms of bifurcation fails to grasp the interdependence of rehabilitation – re-education with social dangerousness. By retaining a theoretical centrality for the criminal justice system it risks assuming the self legitimation of the latter as a description of its actual operations. The metaphor of bifurcation imputes to the criminal justice system the production of processes which in reality have their origins elsewhere. By accentuating the separation between the criminal justice system and other systems which produce control, the metaphor fails to grasp the residual nature of the category of social dangerousness and identifies its origin within the criminal justice system itself. Bifurcation is rather the creature of the crisis of the welfare system, and its origins should be looked for within the 'circuit' of welfare agencies. Such a shift in focus implies the adoption of a different model of interpretation. When viewed from the standpoint of the agencies of welfare and social services the metaphor of a 'circuit' (trans-institutionalism) seems rather more adequate than that of bifurcation to come to terms with the universe of control producing institutions.

Circuit is a metaphor which underlines not only the interdependence but also the continual interchange between the criminal justice system and the system of welfare and social services together with their functioning through a process of reciprocal referral. This model assumes nevertheless that the criminal justice system functions as the point of arrival and classification, as the indispensable support of the entire circuit and as the producer of models of custodial and segregating control in the last instance.

Such a circuit is anything but peaceful. It is useful to retain from the bifurcation metaphor the notion of tensions existing between the different modes of control. It is precisely these tensions, plus those internal to welfare agencies themselves, which produce social dangerousness. It is necessary first of all to remember that the welfare agencies are primarily concerned with the redistribution of resources. The production of control is secondary and is a by-product of the disciplinary and normative aspects of the distribution process. As far as welfare agencies are concerned, their role in the pacification and normalisation of conflict, in the management of hardship and social disturbance and in the translation of these into problems of individual pathology, is inextricably bound up with the role of these agencies in the production and diffusion of social rights. It is this latter function which is their primary and legitimating one, taking the form of responses to needs. Such needs are of course themselves administratively predefined by the welfare system itself which then interacts with the needs as it has defined them. The more rigid the predefinition of needs, the more problematic and contradictory the effects of interaction with them.

There are therefore many factors which determine in practice the operation of the normalising role of welfare agencies. From the planning, formation and implementation of policies to the interaction between the services they comprise (Micheli 1986), between these agencies themselves and the criminal justice system, between services and their clients, such operation is the outcome of conflicts and negotiations. Social dangerousness is one of the possible products of these processes: whose interface is however a new type of subjectivity.

Because dangerousness comes to be that which remains, resists or falls through the net of welfare agencies, all that which cannot be managed by or is irreducible to the operative rules of these agencies, many such phenomena appear as 'neglect'. Neglect has however two faces: on one side it indicates a failure of the system and therefore forms the basis of a critique of welfare policy, on the other hand, it denotes a site of formless resistance to institutional intervention. Inasmuch as neglect is not only the result of the inadequacies of the system but also of the non-manageability of problems, it tends to present itself in the form of 'social disturbance'. In this form neglect becomes interpreted as social dangerousness.

If neglect directs attention to the responsibilities of welfare agencies and evokes a care model, social dangerousness directs attention to the criminal justice system and evokes the model of custody. When the emphasis is on neglect, social dangerousness is re-configured in therapeutic terms appropriate to demands for, and experiments in, a type of social control backed up by custodial measures of a 'community service' type. Such strategies seek legitimacy through an appeal to the right of the individual to receive care and the duty of the state to provide it, even against the wishes of the client (I refer to the debate on drug dependency, obligatory cure, the therapeutic community). When, on the other hand, the accent is on social dangerousness, then neglect acquires a quality indissolubly associated with lifestyles, attitudes and cultures (Pizzorno 1986). Gypsies and ethnic minorities are perceived and defined as socially dangerous precisely on those grounds. The fact of living or coming from socially and culturally deprived areas, with a high rate of crime, like some neighbourhoods of Palermo and Naples, is also associated with social dangerousness. Such characterisations of neglect lead to demands for security of which the criminal justice system is the focus.

There is also another way to look at the dialectic neglect–dangerousness. These two terms can be understood, for example, as moves in a conflict or conflicts between welfare agencies and the criminal justice system and between the entire circuit of institutions and the public. In the first case the absence of custodial solutions on the part of welfare agencies may be used by these agencies themselves to justify the neglect of what they define as social disturbance and which is, as such, referred back to the criminal justice system. In the second case the situation is more complex. The boundaries between neglect and dangerousness are subtle and mobile, and the public uses both terms, often simultaneously, in conflicts with the welfare agencies, as in the cases when neglect is denounced as the source of social dangerousness, or when social services are required to intervene for reasons of social defence (see, for example the struggles around the issues of drug dependency and mental illness).

DANGEROUS OR TREATABLE: A NON-RIGID ALTERNATIVE

The interpretation of social dangerousness discussed above makes possible an understanding of the dynamics of social control which grasps the process of change and relocation of conflicts.

The centrality of the crime issue or rather, as we shall see in later chapters, the translation of the crime issue into a penal issue in much Anglo-Saxon sociology and critical criminology, led to flattened scenarios, often reflective of those depicted by much 1960s sociology. The pessimistic interpretation I referred to above sees the exit from the criminal justice system (in Anglo-Saxon legislation) of certain crimes without victims – abortion, homosexuality, prostitution, drug dependency, some forms of juvenile delinquency – no longer as a success for the politics of decriminalisation associated with the left during the 1960s,[14] but as the outcome of conservative policies geared towards the pathologisation of conflicts. From this point of view, the criminal justice system appears at least as the site where conflicts are recognised as such and where the individuals involved in them retain the status of actors whose motivations have to be taken into consideration.[15] The 'back to justice' movement is inspired by a concern with respect for civil liberties, seen as threatened by rehabilitative models of response to social problems. The return to retributionist models may then be invoked in the name of the protection of the rights of individuals, and criminal justice may then be seen as the site where the motivations of actors are taken seriously instead of being reduced to mere expressions of pathologies.

However, the return to the focus on punishment which was evident during the 1980s in the United States (and in a different way in Italy) was predicated not so much on the protection of civil liberties as on the necessity of social defence, and it resulted in making irrelevant not only the sociocultural causes of criminality but also the individual motivations of offenders. (See the so-called right wing realist criminologists discussed in Platt, Tagaki 1978.)

According to Cohen (1983), the couplet dangerousness–social defence signifies precisely the return to behaviourist models indicating a significant slippage from the centrality of the mind to the centrality of the body. This slippage, a result of the crisis of the rehabilitative ideology, is functional to a politics of crime whose realistic objective (according to its supporters) is not the elimination or reduction of the causes of crime, nor the re-education and rehabilitation of the offender, but that of rendering the criminals (naturally those which manage to get caught) harmless. According to Cohen, this politics justifies itself precisely in terms of the necessity of social defence to confront dangerousness, and focuses on disadvantaged social groups while the question of motivation and therefore of the themes of re-education and rehabilitation retain their relevance as regards middle class deviance. In contrast to the 'back to justice' liberals, Cohen argues that some attention to 'consciousness' and therefore some recognition of the status of the offender as actor is retrievable rather in the universe of therapy and other services directed towards the 'monitoring' of the middle classes than in the return to punishment to which socially disadvantaged groups are subject.

In Italy, however, a rather more confused picture presents itself (and it is at least hypothesisable that the adoption of a conceptual starting point de-centred from the penal system would to some extent give different results when applied to the United States). In Italy the psychiatric welfare system is a composite area characterised by the coexistence and interaction of public, semi-public and private services, the potential clients of which are not easily distinguishable on the basis of sociological characteristics and who in effect circulate between institutions (presumably with different strategies, depending on different personal resources). Besides, if we conceive of social dangerousness (and social defence) as the combined residual product of the 'circuit' and as a move in conflict, the two models of control, body and mind, incapacitation and intervention on social causes and individual motivations, present themselves as inextricably connected. Each interfaces with, or provides a continuous constraint and challenge to, the other both within the penal and inside the system of welfare and social services. Certainly they do not identify sociologically distinct populations (see De Leonardis 1988).

SOCIAL DANGEROUSNESS, SUBJECTIVISATION AND THE IMPUTATION OF RESPONSIBILITY

I would like to pick up again in conclusion the question of the relationship between subjectivisation and social dangerousness. It seems to me in fact to exemplify the dynamics and contradictions of an imputation of responsibility initiated by the welfare state. That which becomes constructed as dangerousness is precisely that which presents itself as ungovernable and untreatable. The untreatability (or intractability) can, as I have already argued, be thematised as a deficiency on the part of the institutions or as a characteristic of the phenomenon itself. In both cases an imputation of responsibility is in play. In the first case the ideology of welfare is carried to its extreme consequences and becomes a weapon in the conflict with the welfare agencies themselves: if all problems are in principle treatable then those which are not treated cannot any longer be seen as naturally resistant to treatment but rather as the result of inefficiency, inactivity, perversity, or bad faith on the part of the responsible institutions. In the second case untreatability is constructed as a form of voluntary resistance. This construction is the means by which the agencies of welfare defend and legitimate the boundaries of their proper competences. Untreatability is constructed as the subjective refusal of treatment.

These are the themes which social dangerousness conveys today. Indeed, the conflict among the agencies and between agencies and clients is played out inside the culture and politics of welfare. The welfare agencies are not free to pronounce a condition as naturally non-treatable without other agencies and/or the clients presenting the intractability of that same condition as a challenge, a failure on the part of the agency which has so defined it.

Resistance to, and unavailability for, treatment denote figures of danger different from the traditional, overdetermined, ones, typically the mad, the habitual delinquent, the innate criminal. For the penal system the new figures are the terrorist, the mafiosi, the 'violent' criminal. They have their correlates in less explicitly menacing figures, less conscious enemies, on the welfare side, throughout that area defined, on one side by the failure of the agencies and on the other by the unanswered demands and claims of the clients. It is the context of conflict which comes to define the area of dangerousness: an area associated not so much with one particular condition as with the shifting movements of the conflict itself. But in this sense the area of dangerousness takes on precisely that degree of subjective autonomy which makes it unpredictable, ungovernable, and thus in certain ways, antagonistic.

DICHOTOMIES

I wish to challenge, and this is a constant theme in this book, the productivity of dichotomies such as body and mind, rehabilitation and punishment, criminal justice and welfare, freedom and responsibility, civil liberties and social rights, for understanding contemporary policies of social control. I want to avoid what seems to me to have been a constant theme in 'progressive' assessments of these policies and even more in 'progressive' evaluations of welfare policies and their present crisis: namely, the oscillation between advocacy of welfare measures aimed at intervening in the causes of social problems and denunciation of these measures themselves as oppressive and erosive of individual freedoms. Such oscillation is translated, when social control policies are the main target, into periodic bursts of enthusiasm for delegalisation, de-institutionalisation, etc., rapidly succeeded by cries for a return to the rule of law.

I will also argue that these two positions are indicative of different ways of conceiving the status of the individual actor and of her relationships with 'society', which in turn give rise to different ways of theorising the relationship between individual, social and political responsibilities.

I will argue in the succeeding chapters that what we are confronting today is indeed a complex and controversial return of the problematics of the actor, and his/her rights, in opposition to that of the 'social system', and its structural contradictions. But this return occurs in the context of a developed welfare culture, in which 'needs' are increasingly translated into social rights, which in this guise are at the basis of new demands, new conflicts, and new forms of organisation.

The institutional uncertainty that is the outcome not only of the crisis of welfare, but also of the way this crisis is interpreted by institutional and social actors, is a rich field for the investigation of the meaning and direction of contemporary social control policies. But such institutional uncertainty can be grasped only if we get rid of dichotomous grids, and use instead models which permit us to see the connections (and therefore the conflicts) between different institutions and agencies and between institutions and agencies and social actors. Conversely, such exploration of social control policies may also become an instrument with which to interrogate the actual status of social and political actors. I will argue that what is at the core of present social policies and political questions is precisely the issue of responsibility. But this issue can and is posed in different ways. It can be constructed to signify the return to the scene of abstract actors merely endowed with 'negative' rights or the appearance on the scene of 'embedded' actors who require a different understanding of the relationship between freedom and responsibility.

As I address these themes from the point of view of the 'criminal question' (an unusual – admittedly decentred – site from which to look at them, and also an unusual use of the criminal question itself), I retain the notion of social control precisely for its ambiguity, e.g. for the possibilities it offers to escape from dichotomous grids.

2 Studying the 'criminal question'
The object of criminology and the responsibility of the criminologist

There is today a widespread questioning of the notion of responsibility. The issues to which this term refers are many and diverse and it is important not to confuse them. In this chapter I will attempt to confront the re-emergence of the theme of responsibility within the bodies of knowledge concerned with inquiry into the nature of crime. Such re-emergence is, as I shall seek to show, related to socio-cultural changes of vast importance, of which the crisis in these disciplines themselves is only one, marginal, aspect. This crisis refers to the development of a field of institutional uncertainty which one tries to confront – in this as well as in other cases – by means of a not always well thought out 'ethical' vocabulary. The question of responsibility is, on the other hand, strictly connected, as will be seen, to ways of defining, conceiving of, and studying the so-called criminal question.

THE PARADOX OF RESPONSIBILITY

Responsibility is a moral (philosophical) question, and it refers to the consequences of an action to which someone can respond. That implies first of all a de-naturalised context. It is not necessary that the result of a certain action is conceived of as intentionally willed: it is, however, necessary that the subject of that action is seen as capable of acting intentionally, and the action itself is seen as one of the alternatives available to the subject. To speak of an 'objective' responsibility is not to impute the consequences of a certain action to the conscious design of an actor, but implies nevertheless that the actor ought to and can respond to them. The consequences of an action can be unintended, unpredicted, unwilled, but in order to speak of responsibility, such consequences have precisely to be referable to an action (or a series of actions) instead of to events seen as natural or to behaviour viewed as entirely determined by instinct. That means that 'responsibility' can only exist in a de-naturalised universe. We live precisely in a universe which is increasingly de-naturalised, not unlike those so-called primitives for whom no event was independent of human action (Douglas and Wildavsky 1983). In one way or another all the 'world views' which have dominated the last two centuries have contributed to such de-naturalisation. The result has been the extension of the field of responsibility. Secularisation and the supremacy of scientific knowledge, far from resulting in the domination of a naturalism neutral with respect to values as regards human relations and relations between human beings and their natural and social environment, has led on the contrary to the consideration of such relations and environment as the product of human action. The extension of the human capacity to intervene in the social and natural circumstances of life, and the consciousness of this power, imply the multiplication and diversification of questions concerning objectives, means, effects and the legitimacy of intervention itself. Nature becomes socialised and politicised at the same time that the social comes to be studied *as if* it were 'natural'. What I want to argue is that even (indeed, above all) the nineteenth-century positivist paradigm not only did not negate, but on the contrary reinforced and multiplied, the possibilities for the extension of the sphere of responsibility. If the determinism of the linear link between cause and effect in the scientific knowledge of nature does not admit subjective inference and excludes nature itself from the horizon of ends and values, it permits and indeed is oriented towards, the extension of human control over nature.

The same link, as a key concept for the interpretation of the social, produces strategies for the purposive control of society and constitutes actors involved in projects of conscious social change. Extreme naturalistic reductivism is in reality never a dominant position and never really implies the rejection of intervention. At the most it results in a paradox: the lack of the capacity for responsibility on the part of some individuals implies that others assume the responsibility for counteracting them. The awareness of a (presumed) determinism linking certain biological characteristics to certain types of social behaviour can only, in its turn, imply the political imperative to do something so that the biological causes of negatively valued social behaviour are taken under control or, in the worst case, that the 'bearers' of these characteristics are eliminated. And politics is the site of responsibility. In one sense, the supremacy of the deterministic paradigm, however elaborated, is inextricably bound up with both the assumption of and the imputation of responsibility. Consciousness produces power, but above all it produces the consciousness of power which in its turn implies the imperative to activate power in accordance with a project or goal.

The naturalising gaze both produces politics and is the product of politics. Thus, as an obvious example, the irresponsibility of the criminal lays responsibilities on the criminologist and whoever has to decide how to maintain public order. If the causes of events are understood and knowable, the events themselves become no longer inevitable. And that carries with it the obligation to choose whether or not to allow them to take place.

In another sense the supremacy of the scientific paradigm introduces an explicit debate on the attribution of responsibility, the requisites upon which such attribution ought to, or can, be based and on the (scientifically ascertainable) degrees of human freedom. It is necessary to distinguish between this debate and the general implications and consequences – cultural, political and social – to which the supremacy of the scientific paradigm has given rise (and of which it is a product). The sociological and biological hyper-determinism of certain formulations, approaches and interpretations (within my own field: Skinnerian behaviourism or the continually recurring idea of the criminal as such by nature), not only fails to extinguish but in reality gives sustenance to the socialisation and politicisation of the human universe and hence to the multiplication of questions of responsibility.

The present crisis of the scientistic paradigm, or rather the paradoxes to which scientific and technological innovations have given place, has intensified and made explicit the issues of responsibility and fostered a powerful return of the moral dimension in public discourse. Who decides the boundaries between life and death now that these boundaries have become so uncertain? Who decides when human life begins and when we should start protecting it? and so on.

It is not then only a question of going once more through the history of the scientific and cultural debate on conceptions of the actor, by tracing the boundaries between deterministic and voluntaristic interpretations of human action. This history is permeated with, produced by and itself produces, politics and interventions oriented by projects, new obligations and new rights. And, at times paradoxically, also the consciousness of all this, resulting therefore in new social and political actors, new demands, new conflicts.

It may be pertinent on the other hand to read the history of the scientific debate from a standpoint which problematises the various positions, understanding their interaction with the social and political consequences which they explicitly or implicitly prefigure. It will then be easier to see the changing relationship between attribution and assumption of responsibility, on one hand the meaning assigned to the term itself and on the other how the limits to the field of its imputation may imply an extension of the field of its assumption.

Responsibility has therefore a double face: as a question of *social* responsibility which refers to the causes and functions of social phenomena and as a question of individual responsibility to society and other individuals which refers to the status of actors.

As far as the bodies of knowledge concerned with the investigation of the criminal question in particular are concerned (though an analogous discourse applies to all the social sciences), no discussion of the criteria for the attribution of responsibility to the 'criminal' can avoid a simultaneous discussion of the assumption of responsibility both by the 'criminologist' and by the institutions and individuals who perform the tasks of defining, selecting and administering the criminals themselves. The status of the former is strictly connected to the status of the latter. I say the bodies of knowledge concerned with the investigation of the criminal question (henceforth for brevity grouped under the general term 'criminology') in particular, because these are disciplines which are inextricably bound up with practical and political concerns, and neither have, nor any longer claim, any autonomy with respect to how their object of study is constructed within the logic of concrete institutions, and whose knowledge aims are also immediately aims which are related to or productive of *policies*.

A DE-SUBJECTIFIED SOCIALISATION

The scenario in which we move has been then, for at least two centuries, an increasingly socialised one. I would underline two fundamental components of the culture of our century, of which both the influence and the crisis can aid an understanding of the way in which the theme of responsibility is re-stated today. I refer to Marxism and to what I would term, rather imprecisely, welfare culture (which itself owes much to Marxism), or rather the culture produced by the extension of the welfare state. Both emphasise the historical and social dimension of human existence, proclaiming the social (and therefore historical) nature of 'wrong' – injustice, oppression, illness, poverty, etc. Indeed, as we shall see, it is the very attribution of injustice and oppression which renders problematic social conditions which would otherwise be lived as natural. That which is social is evidently the product, however complex, of human action. It implies a simultaneous imputation and assumption of responsibility. However difficult it is to reconstruct the chain of 'causes' of the present, the assumption is that not only is it possible to do so but that the result takes the form of identifiable actions, of whatever degree of intentionality, which have produced the present situation and to which other actions can counterpose themselves in order to limit, contain or re-orient. The active subjects of these actions, as well as the actions' pace (see Jonas 1984) are differently identified in Marxism and in what I call the 'welfare culture'. But what is analogous, even if more emphasised in Marxism, is that rationality is not so much a property of the single – or the collective – actor, as of the historical process as such. Typically, the actors understand fully what they have done only after they have acted. Their actions are both determined by history (by the consequences of the actions which have preceded them) and are able to intervene in this history itself; the more freely and effectively they do so the more developed is their awareness of the modes of determination. The actors are only in part responsible for what they are but in the process of coming to understand the conditions of their existence, they are increasingly endowed with responsibility for their future. They are therefore neither impotent nor omnipotent.

Yet this status of the limited rationality of the actor, contrasted to a historical process to which full rationality is imputed, has given way, depending on the circumstances, to a formulation in terms of either impotence or omnipotence. Omnipotence takes the form of the revolutionary discontinuity produced by the victorious collective actor, or that of the continuous improvement produced by a plurality of actors (collective or individual) who intervene knowledgeably in the actual conditions of their life. Impotence, by contrast, portrays the revolutionary discontinuity as the product of the rationality of the historical process rather than that of the conscious collective actor; or a scenario where the plurality of 'knowledgeable' actors is swallowed up and hidden within the apparatuses, institutions and systems which become autonomous from the actors and usurp and perfect their wisdom. In this second formulation we have still a socialised universe but one in which the assumption and the attribution of responsibility identifies not actors but rather processes, mechanisms, which are comprehended without reference to their being the product of (intended or unintended) actions.

The recent crisis of the two paradigms involves both versions. The Collective Actor, protagonist of transformation, is fragmented and de-centered and the historical process is revealed as deprived of any intrinsic rationality. The projects of reform and social engineering produce new questions and new problems and their results never correspond to the 'good intentions' of those who formulated them; the institutional 'responses' obey their own logic, apparently indifferent to the demands to which they are supposed to respond and to the efforts of those who work within them.[1]

It is again necessary to distinguish between the scientific and philosophical debate to which this double crisis has given rise, and the analysis of how it has been perceived, theorised and carried into effect in the wider culture. Obviously in this I limit myself to the scientific debate around the issues and problems surrounding 'crime' or what I shall term the criminal question.

CRIMINOLOGIES

By criminology I mean the various bodies of knowledge which go under the (academic) titles of the sociology of deviance, social control, juvenile delinquency, criminal law etc., which deal with various aspects of the 'criminal question'. I defer until later a discussion of the meaning of this concept and what, in my opinion, beyond academic labels, it implies as regards theoretical and methodological issues. Here I would like to briefly trace certain aspects of the history of the study of the criminal question during the last twenty years. My reconstruction is both approximate, and partial, because I am concerned in the present context, only with certain aspects of this history (but see Baratta 1982; Cohen 1985; Faccioli,1984; Pavarini 1981; Pitch 1982).

The debate, overwhelmingly Anglo-Saxon, during the 1960s and the first half of the 1970s can be roughly characterised as dominated by two tendencies. The first, traditional, constructs crime as a taken-for-granted social problem for which the task is to establish the causes by tracing the complex interactions between social, economic, cultural and psychological factors. The problem of crime is indeed a social question, it has its roots in social processes and is to be dealt with as such. But it reveals itself through the 'criminal' behaviour of individuals. As has been noted (see chapter 1) there are at least two principal versions of this tendency: one, so to speak, 'Rooseveltian' in which criminality is seen as a process of normal adaption (*rational with respect to its aims*) to a *structurally* anomic social situation; and a consolidated welfare version, in which criminality is seen as irrational adaption to early pathological interactions (Merton 1971, Parsons 1965, chap. X). Because the first version, even more than the second, in its various formulations has long represented the dominant theoretical understanding and has contributed to the construction of a generalised common sense, it will be convenient to study more closely the way in which it poses the issues of 'responsibility'.

The criminal is neither abnormal nor ill.[2] His[3] actions and motives have to be understood through the same processes as non-criminal behaviour. The problem is displaced therefore onto the status of the actor (it is no accident that the criminal and the deviant occupy such a central place in American sociology: precisely because they offer themselves as material on which to construct the ideal type of actor). The actor is indeed 'rational' but this rationality is 'instrumental' and concerns the choice of efficient means to ends which are given in the cultural system and, through socialisation, internalised in the personality system. From a strictly technical point of view, therefore, the actor is responsible for the consequences of his actions: he knows what he is doing and why. At the same time he is not responsible for his motivations inasmuch as these are culturally defined goals which cannot but have been passively internalised. Neither is he responsible for the fact that, typically for the criminal, he finds himself in a social position which makes it difficult or impossible to act out his motivations in legal or legitimate ways. In this interpretation of criminality there are no 'innocents'. The responsibilities, nevertheless, are differently conceived and emphasised. There is a general political responsibility to intervene to attenuate or eliminate the conditions creating 'anomie'.[4] There are 'local' institutional responsibilities concerning the conditions in a specific situation: a particular district for example. There is the individual responsibility of the offender: but this, compared to the responsibility of 'society', is merely, it might be said, a technical question: a symptom of things not functioning and of the necessity for social and political intervention, both at the social level and at the level of the individual offender, both inside and outside the prison. Hence the limited responsibility of the criminal implies a more extensive, heavy and articulate 'social' responsibility in the dual sense that crime has social 'causes' and that 'society' has therefore the obligation to take responsibility for the consequences of crime and for the removal of its causes.

As far as the second version is concerned, the status of the criminal is equivalent to that of the sick. This means that the criminal cannot be considered responsible for his actions. He has, however, the obligation to collaborate with his own cure (see Parsons 1965, chap. X) and there have to be institutions adequate to cure him. 'Failure' in either respect can result in a pronouncement of the non-retrievability of the offender and/or the rejection as useless of therapeutic oriented strategies of social control.

These two versions of traditional criminology are based on and have contributed to the development of social and penal policies inspired by concepts such as rehabilitation and re-socialisation, and have permeated, in various combinations, the common sense of the agencies created to implement such policies.

The second tendency affirms itself precisely in a context of the consolidated welfare state and, as I have argued in chapter 1, can be interpreted as a critique of the pathologising and de-responsibilising consequences of welfare policies. It constructs the issue of crime as the result of interaction between deviant actions and institutional reactions. Because criminality is seen as the end result of social and institutional processes of social control, the analysis is displaced from the 'causes' of the criminal act to the examination of these processes of interaction. (I refer to the so-called labelling theorists: Becker 1987; Erikson 1962; Kitsuse 1962; Lemert 1951, 1981; and to Goffman 1963, 1968; Matza 1976). My focus here is those aspects of the analysis which found their way into the 'alternative culture' of the 1970s and I leave out of consideration therefore the variety of different ways in which this general approach has been developed.

The focus of this tendency was on one hand the unintended and perverse consequences of social and penal politics with respect to their objectives, and on the other the impotence of the individual actor in the face of apparatuses and mechanisms which impose on him a definition of the situation from which he cannot escape. The theme of perverse consequences emphasises the limits of rationality in the control of social events and forms the basis of a critique of the illusion of omnipotence. On the other hand, the actor is constructed as locally competent in the sense that what he does and how he perceives and defines himself is the normal result of interactive processes in specific situations. The consequences of action are therefore attributable to a plurality of actors involved in defining the situation. In the case of the 'criminal' the consequences to be analysed are not so much those that result from the illegal action itself, as those which derive from the institutional reaction to it. It is the latter which constructs the 'problem', by amplifying, fixing, and reshaping it in accordance with the prevailing modes of operation of the institutions – constructing it, for example, as a medical or penal issue – and by stabilising and reproducing the characteristics of the actors in terms of deviant careers, habitual recidivism etc. It is this institutional reaction, then, which is 'responsible' for the problem, not so much in terms of having to take responsibility for it as in the sense of being responsible for the negative consequences of the construction of the problem as such.

There are at least two aspects to be underlined here. Analyses in terms of perverse consequences, though they have continually given rise to a 'pessimism', which takes, as we shall see, different forms in both 'right' and 'left', have also been the result of attempts to reclaim islands of freedom in a society seen as increasingly colonised and administered. The distrust of the plan, the large centralised institution, the totalizing project, is articulated in the traditional language of American liberalism: the individual against the large bureaucracy (see Cassano 1971). But such distrust gives expression also to the new experience of a contradiction between the claims of a totalizing institutional control and greater possibilities for the autonomous definition of self. These analyses arise within the welfare state and give value to its economic and cultural resources. They put into focus the intelligence and the competence of the individual actor. It is to the actor's communicative and reflexive capacities that a resolution of the controversies and conflicts are entrusted, such as to be as close as possible to the lived experience of the actors themselves, be they employees of the agencies of social control or their clients.[5] Thus only by means of the deconstruction of established rigid, totalizing, definitions (and therefore interventions), irrelevant to local situations, is it possible to restore to the actors the responsibility for their own actions.

The interface of all this is the construction of the actor (the deviant, the criminal) as victim: not so much of social injustice but of the power/ knowledge of institutions. The conflict emphasised is that between the individual actor (the citizen, bearer of civil rights) and 'the system'.

During the 1970s, in England, in Germany, in Italy[6] and also the United States, this tendency came to converge with an orientation variously influenced by Marxism. So-called critical criminology assumed different forms and outcomes in relation to the various political cultures and conjunctures in individual countries (see Baratta 1982; Greenberg 1977, 1981; NDC 1980; NDC/CSE 1979; Taylor, Walton, Young 1975; Pitch 1983; Platt, Takagi 1981; and the journals: *La Questione Criminale* in Italy, *Crime and Social Justice* in the United States, and *Déviance et Société* in France). It is certainly not correct to see, as some have (see Young 1986), critical criminology as a coherent and unified paradigm. What I intend to examine here are some of its themes which, during the 1970s, passed into the culture of the 'left' and even into the common sense of the agencies of social control – though more on the level of what was talked about rather than what was acted upon (see Cohen 1983), and yet influencing the objectives and the self-perceptions of practitioners.

The criminal question was conceived as the result of a double selection: an initial selection at the level of actions to be criminalised (or of the juridical goods to be protected); the second operating on the level of the individuals to whom to attribute the status of criminals. The two selections responded to definite needs of domination and its reproduction. Criminality was conceived as a 'negative good', unequally but not arbitrarily distributed. Members of the lower classes are selected as criminals, both because criminal law is constructed to take care of the interests of the upper classes, and because of the functioning of the operative logic and concrete practice of the agencies of social control.

This interpretation linked the processes identified by the labelling theorists to a particular configuration of power, associated with a particular socio-economic system. The consequences of these processes, therefore, were not perverse in relation to their objectives: on the contrary, they were entirely consistent, if not with the explicit intentions of legislators, with the implicit, hidden, logic of power. It was therefore a question of laying bare this logic, of showing how the criminal question is reproduced unaltered whatever current policies define and administer it, if the basic mechanisms, the structure of power, distribution of socio-economic resources are left untouched. The problematic nature of the acts selected as criminal, not only for the collectivity but also for those who commit them, was not negated:

they were read as 'symptoms' of hardship, as 'necessitated' by needs, or as distorted expressions of conflicts. The criminal was a double victim: of unjust social conditions, and of an unjust criminal justice system.

The criminal becomes here both the symbol of oppression and consequently the standard bearer of revolt. In both cases however, the offender is only partially responsible for what he does. His action, perfectly rational in the technical sense, reveals itself as the inadequate, and in some ways irrational, response to his situation. To the limited rationality of the criminal there corresponds the hidden rationality of the process of domination, whose dynamics continue unseen, despite the 'good intentions' of the reformers.

This interpretation allowed for a variety of political proposals. Even if the 'optimal' solution to the criminal question was entrusted to general social and political changes, intervention at the level of penal and social policy was not rejected. Specific projects often suffered from this tension between 'reformist' and 'revolutionary' aims, tension which was often destined to dissolve into pessimism. While such projects took into account what they saw as not so much the failures as the necessary consequences of penal and social policies in the welfare state, they situated themselves, however, within the context created by these policies and aimed to diminish, soften and even to subordinate measures of social control, such as depenalisation, decriminalisation and decarceration, to the goal of increasing the cultural and economic resources available for the individual 'criminal' and of the collectivity of which he formed part.

The scenario changed considerably over the next fifteen years. The assumptions behind both the expansion of welfare state measures on the one hand and the possibility of revolutionary transformation on the other entered into a crisis. Before describing how this double crisis was reflected in the politics of crime, I would like to make some general remarks on the criminologies of the 1960s and 1970s. These criminologies share both an attribution of rationality to the actor and a recognition of the limitations of this rationality. The consequences of illegal actions are determined by a complex of interactions and/or circumstances which put them outside the conscious control of those who undertake them. Rather, they refer to the actions of those institutions and actors which enter into these interactions from a position of power or which have contributed to the production of these circumstances. The key interactions to be studied are therefore those between the 'criminal' and these institutions and actors rather than those between the 'criminal' and his 'victims'. Criminal actions in this context are seen as examples or symptoms of a general economic, social, cultural and political condition characterised by domination by one class of another (or others). The status of the 'criminal' is a particular case of the status of the 'oppressed'. The nature of this oppression changes between different criminologies with the result that not only are different strategies held to be necessary to combat it, but different subjects of the struggle are identified. However in all of them there is the conviction of the dual task of criminology: on one hand the production of programmes for political and institutional intervention, on the other the deconstruction of the criminal question, that is, the theoretical and practical dismantling of the knowledges and institutions which have constructed it.

The criminologies of the 1960s and 1970s contributed to a perception of the omnipotence of *collective* actors. Because, if one attributes to the criminal only a limited rationality, and to the agencies of control an indirect rationality, independent of conscious projects and intentions, it is the collective actor, either of the reformist or revolutionary variety, that is seen to be, at least potentially, in a position to develop comprehensive solutions and to pursue them consciously.

It is precisely this latter assumption which has entered most deeply into crisis – whether as the fragmentation and dispersal of the collective historical subject, as the failure of large-scale reforms, or as the disappearance of the idea of the intrinsic rationality of the historical process. It is within this horizon that the question of responsibility resurfaces. It signals in the first place a new interest in ethical questions – or rather a translation of political questions into ethical questions which has at least in part been due to the increased perception of the dramatic limitations of political rationality on one hand and of the perverse consequences of technological development on the other. But as far as we are concerned here, the resurrection of the debate on responsibility relates also to a different deployment and perception of conflicts, to a change in the self comprehension of the actors. Criminological and socio-juridical literature has both reflected and attempted to interpret these changes. But by starting, for the most part, only from the results of changes which specifically focus on penal politics and social control, such literature usually reflects a lack of reflexivity and consciousness, which are not least among the present discomforts of criminologists. Let us now look at the current state of criminology.

VARIETIES OF REALISM

Criminology as epidemiology

Three different approaches compete in the area of contemporary debate outside Italy. Of course, this is a simplification because many other positions exist. Indeed the characteristic of the present debate is really that of the co-presence of different tendencies increasingly less clearly locatable as unified currents. Nevertheless, the three approaches to be described here are adequate to the task of describing the main ways with which the crisis previously underlined is being reflected within criminology.

Two of these approaches define themselves as 'realist'. This self-definition is polemical. It stands to signify both that the problems of criminality (we shall see presently what they are) are to be considered as 'real', true, serious, and that the intention is to contribute to the creation of projects and measures which are realistic in the triple sense of non-utopian, implementable, and adequate to their purpose.

The first type of realism, variously elaborated, has strongly influenced, if not the concrete policies, at least the debate around the criminal question in the United States (see Platt, Takagi 1977; Greenberg, Humphries 1981). It has been understood as perfectly consistent with Reaganite strategies aimed at the reduction of the welfare state and, more generally, as the product of an increasing tendency to the transformation of politics into administration. A right-wing realism, conservative, oriented to the defence of public order, then, which is however no stranger to the recovery of traditional liberal themes.[7] Retributivist politics, in fact, are supported as a response to a problem characterised in terms of 'social dangerousness' (see also chapter 1).

The policies inspired by strategies of rehabilitation are denounced as useless and costly. While 'left' critics focus on the therapeutic and totalitarian tendencies of rehabilitation, this type of 'realism' proclaims the uselessness of the rehabilitative model is evidenced by the increasing rates of crime, recidivism etc. What is advocated therefore is a return to, and an intensification of, the strategy of retribution, argued for in terms of both its reduced costs and its effect in terms of deterrence. The politics of 'just deserts' is not only augured by conservatives: during the early 1970s it was at the centre of a package of recommendations from the American Friends Service Committee Working Party (1971), a liberal organisation concerned with the defence of juridical guarantees and civil rights seen as threatened by measures which increased the area of discretion, arbitrariness and inequality in the implementation of penalties.[8] What is common to the critics of the 'right' and the 'left' is the conception of the criminal as a conscious actor. Where the latter insist that the penal response be respectful of the personality of the criminal, rejecting, that is, the project of reforming it – and that this response is rather a response to the action and not a response to the author – the former re-emphasises the notion of deterrence. It makes no sense and is anyway impossible to change the criminals: but they can be discouraged by the threat of severe, certain and swiftly imposed punishment. The left attribute to punishment the purpose of 'moral' retribution for wrong (just deserts). The right see the purpose of punishment as that of 'terrorising', but, once imposed, that of neutralising, or incapacitating (see, for example, von Hirsch 1975; Van den Haag 1975; Wilson 1975).

The criminal question becomes once more the problem of criminals. But the motivations and social conditions producing 'criminals' are no more of interest. The 'causes' of crime, long at the centre of analysis and debate, sought in psychology, in social conditions or in the working of the agencies of control, cease to be the object of inquiry. The task of the criminologist is the identification of measures adequate to contain and limit the danger constituted by criminality.

However any interventionist project implies some theory of the nature and conditions in which crime arises, and typical of these realists is eclecticism, or an assemblage of different theories with a decisive preference towards those which insist on psychological, biological or even genetic factors (see Wilson, Herrnstein 1985).

There is an apparent contradiction in these approaches. On one hand they insist on the existence of crime as the result of an individual choice, independent of the social and cultural context and hence characteristic of individuals in some way oriented to 'wrong' (in these 'theories' obviously, crime regains an ontological status: that which is illegal is so because universally disapproved of and therefore wrong in itself). On the other hand this orientation can be scientifically ascertained and controlled, it is not randomly distributed. This contradiction is in reality functional with respect to two objectives. While it can be said that 'society' is not responsible for crime (and therefore that reparative or reformative measures are senseless) it is also claimed that 'society' can scientifically fight it. Here eclecticism has free range in furnishing suggestions for different policies, all equally legitimated by a discourse in terms of social defence or the protection of order.

Deterrence and incapacitation are seen as the solutions to a problem which, while not being socially caused, is not randomly distributed in society. The category of social dangerousness becomes central once again (see Bottoms 1977; Mauri 1988) though now deprived of its traditional characteristics (see chapter 1). It no longer describes a criminality anchored in biological characteristics[9] but rather denotes the co-presence of a multiplicity of factors signifying 'risk'. Decisions regarding the amount and type of punishment for example, come to depend on the social dangerousness of the offender formulated as an estimate of the probability of his/her continuing in his criminal activity, derived from various elements such as sex, age, ethnic group, family background, education and employment, measure of intelligence etc. The risk is statistically measurable, and the task of the criminologist becomes that of identifying the categories of individuals at risk. Thus criminology as epidemiology.

Epidemiologist and/or administrator, the realist criminologist is above all involved in a polemic against the philosophies of the welfare state. His/her proposals for intervention, unaffected by references to motivations and causes (s/he is neither interested in 'curing' the criminal nor acting on the causes of crime), accord with and reinforce a common sense originating from the unkept promises of welfare: society is in no way involved, criminals are such because they choose to be so (or are such by nature). In the wider culture the conception of the actor as overdetermined by social structure (which is a perverse consequence of the philosophies of welfare) seems to be replaced, particularly among some social groups, by the rediscovery of individual guilt, wickedness out of choice or by nature, all of which call for a severe, punitive and incapacitating response. This exigency can certainly be understood as a symptom of a widespread unease, an increasing sense of social insecurity, whose roots are many and varied. Another interpretation is however possible, as I shall show later on.

The criminologist as reformer

The so-called new left realism, in its programmatic formulations predominantly British,[10] sees itself as the repentant offspring of critical criminology. Like all such progeny it was overwhelmingly preoccupied, at least initially, to distance itself from its mother, towards whom it did not spare harsh criticisms. Some of these criticisms, apart from an animosity which drove left realists to indiscriminately mix the good with the bad, are pertinent, but above all serve as an indicator of what has changed.

The English left realists (see Lea and Young 1984; Matthews, Young 1986; Young 1986) criticise one of the consequences to which, in their opinion, radical approaches have led, particularly on the left, namely, that it is not crime that is the problem, but the mode of reacting to 'crime'. This has led criminologists in a flight from aetiology towards the elysian fields of the critique of ideology, or at best to the sociology of criminal law. But an escape from aetiology, according to the realists, is also a renunciation of reforms, of knowledge for change, of contributing to the 'solution' of problems. It means a convergence in fact with administrative criminology and similar tendencies. Understanding, an indispensable ingredient of reformist politics, implies therefore, according to the left realists, research into the causes – of crime rather than of the criminal question – because it is crime which is first of all the 'problem'. It is precisely here that the left realists distance themselves from critical criminology – accusing the latter of an idealistic refusal to recognise that crime is above all a problem for the poor and the marginalised, where it arises and where for the most part it takes place. This recognition is accompanied by a new strategy of attention to the 'victims' of crime. According to the left realists the criminologist must 'take seriously people's needs', and that means taking on board questions of security and social defence to which these needs give rise.

In reality such a programme hides a contradiction, as I have argued elsewhere (Pitch 1986). Listening to the 'needs of the people' is in fact a selective process. Only those needs which correspond to the strategy of reforms which the criminologist already has in mind are heard. On the one hand, that is, it is assumed that 'needs' may be directly and – literally – drawn from the demands of 'people'[11] and on the other that such needs be recognised to the extent to which they correspond to the projects of the criminologist-reformer. The victims, in this programme, have an uncertain status. First of all, they are such independently of the fact that they define or perceive themselves as, or act as, victims.[12] But especially, they are endowed with authority and consciousness only as the definers of the problem – an authority and consciousness which is in fact negated when it comes to the formulation of 'solutions'.

A reformist politics such as that formulated by the left realists cannot escape from these contradictions. The project, the plan, the solution, are results prefigured in an analytical paradigm in which criminal behaviour proceeds from social causes (poverty, discrimination, unemployment, etc.) mediated by the subjective perception of 'relative deprivation'. Clearly, and not by chance, left realism resurrects elements of social democratic analysis and strategy, augmenting them with a cultural and subjective dimension which acts as an intermediary between poverty and 'criminality'.

This return to a Mertonian analytical and political perspective reflects unease at the pessimism characterising the current situation. Repressive policies towards crime augured by conservatives and the refusal to formulate policies on the part of radicals, are different responses to the same thing: the 'failure' of the policies of rehabilitation and resocialisation – for conservatives mere costly illusions, and for radicals instruments which widen the scope of institutional intervention, and pathologise conflicts.

While such a return to Merton does not escape the aporias already discussed for its model, it meets with further contradictions when it claims to put the standpoint of the victim at the centre of the preoccupations of the criminologist and of the policies which s/he advocates. In the Mertonian model, the implicit standpoint from which to look at the issue of crime was 'society' in general. Here, on the other hand, crime has a double status: it is at the same time an illegal act and what some social groups consider as harm. The new realists propose themselves as the interpreters of the 'true needs' of social groups whom they consider to be oppressed, exploited and marginalised. It is precisely the standpoint of such groups that they claim to adopt when they proclaim as 'real' the problems which these groups construct as such. These are the 'real' victims, doubly victimised by their social conditions and by crime. To the interaction between 'society' and the criminal is added that between the criminal and his victims. This nevertheless implies a choice which remains unacknowledged. The criminologist-reformer adopts *some* points of view, and since s/he attributes to them a strong reality status on the basis of their belonging to oppressed groups s/he moves within a theoretical horizon which firstly, assumes that there exists a cognitive device for the unambiguous identification of the 'oppressed' apart from the self-identification of the actors concerned and secondly, assumes that the point of view voiced by the oppressed is 'true', as a literal translation of their 'real' needs and, further, that it is naturally 'progressive' – presumably because it is in agreement with some types of teleologically oriented historical rationality.

I will not dwell on the aporias of this approach and of the policies inspired by it.[13] Instead I would like to emphasise its consequences for the issue of responsibility. In the case of both critical and 'reformist' criminologies, the reintroduction of the victims (of crime) into the argument implies a focus on those consequences produced by the actions of certain individuals on the lives of certain others. There is thus at this level a localisation of the attribution of responsibility, which is however frustrated by the claim of the criminologist to confer the status of truth on the victim's perceptions. Thus we have two rather limited rationalities (those of the offender and the victim) and one absolute one (that of the realist criminologist). The criminal offender is responsible for his actions, but acts on the basis of a perception of the situation which in its turn has roots in particular social situations. He is, however, not to be seen as 'determined' by the latter, emphasise the left realists (seeing such a hypothesis as the basis of the failure of social democratic policies). However, since the realists provide neither a theory of the personality nor a theory of action of their own, their invocation of relative deprivation as a connecting link between social conditions and behaviour can only be understood along the lines that we have already seen in Merton's theory of anomie. Finally, the victim – or rather a certain category of victim – is certainly in a position, and indeed is the only subject who is entitled to define the problem, but not to identify the solution unless s/he possesses the same theoretical-political model as the criminologist.

It is, in short, the latter who is the repository of a knowledge which puts her/him in a position to choose the viewpoints of the correct victims. Such knowledge is therefore constructed around a theoretical-political model in which 'causes' and 'actors' interpretations' are in reality inferred from and adjusted to the 'solutions' that the model itself prefigures. It transpires once again that the attribution of 'limited' responsibility to the criminal implies the assumption of a full responsibility on the part of the criminologist. Here however, the 'limitations' of the criminal do not call forth simply a politics of rehabilitation. The amelioration of the social and cultural situations producing criminality does not exclude the criminal justice response. In fact the latter is not only often demanded by the victims in its role of providing protection and compensation, but is also legitimate as a response which takes account of and confirms the non-pathological, non-irrational, nature of the motivations for criminal acts. By comparison with the 'true' victims, criminal offenders are 'victims' only in part. They are by no means innocent.

THE ABOLITIONISTS: CRIMINOLOGY AS DEMYSTIFICATION

At the opposite pole to the realists, at least in the declared intentions of both camps, are the so-called abolitionists. This tendency, for the most part European, with a predominance in Northern Europe (Christie 1985; Hulsman 1982, 1983; Mathiesen 1974, 1983; Scheerer 1983; and for an Italian discussion, Marconi 1983; Pavarini 1985), carries the labelling model to its conclusion. Briefly, abolitionists maintain that 'crime' is not only an arbitrarily imposed label, but one which in reality only serves to conceal and aggravate conflicts, expropriating them from the participants. They do not contest the existence of problematic situations, but contest the adequacy of the response in terms of criminal justice. They maintain, on the contrary, that such a response, beginning with the imposition of the label of crime on certain acts and conflicts, of itself constitutes a problem more serious than the acts and the conflicts which it attempts to resolve. The criminologist has the task of demonstrating this thesis, that is, of revealing the real functions of the system of criminal justice and of describing its perverse consequences. If left realism implies a social democratic politics with the typical emphasis on projects of reform, the politics of abolitionism are more consistent with 'movementism' 'green', vaguely anarchist politics (see Marconi 1983), where the resolution of conflicts is entrusted to mechanisms and processes, of and in the 'community' where they take place. Also in this approach the victims assume a central role. They are seen as expropriated and ignored by the criminal justice system. The abolition of the latter would therefore produce a new and different prota-gonism on the part of victims. Offenders and victims would be put in a position to resolve their 'conflicts' personally in a process of face to face communication in which the 'real' problems of both would retain their concreteness and meaningfulness. The question of the causes of crime – or rather of problems and conflicts which are so labelled – is put in paren-thesis. The criminologist is not directly interested in it, being rather employed in a project of deconstruction of the symbolic and discursive output of the criminal justice system, which is at the same time a project of construction of a community of reasonable actors. The interest in causes, notwithstanding the Marxist origin of many abolitionists, would be inconsistent with a hermeneutic theoretical programme which characterises, more or less explicitly, the abolitionist discourse. Critical of ideology and at the same time involved in the construction of communitarian relations, the abolitionist criminologist oscillates, in a way not altogether unlike her/his left realist 'adversaries', between libertarianism and pedagogy. Whilst the left realists decide that the real problems are what (certain) 'people' say they are, the abolitionists, while they restore to the 'victims' the status of protagonists, assume *de facto* the task of explaining to the victims what the real problems are.

The abolitionists' actor, whether victim or 'criminal', is infinitely reasonable: s/he is capable of assuming responsibility. S/he can and must be put in a position to recognise and deal with the consequences of his/her own actions and thereby directly control the situation. This is possible if the bureaucratic and impersonal structures can be prevented from intervening in the situation and expropriating the participants.

IS THE CRIMINAL QUESTION A PROBLEM OF CRIMINAL JUSTICE?

The problem of what is the criminal question and of how it is constructed by criminological theories, is (as will be seen later), central for an understanding of how the question of responsibility is posed.

In contrast to the 1960s sociologies, critical criminology, abolitionism and the two realisms, in common with so called traditional (clinical, positivist) criminology, allocate a central role to the criminal justice system. This centrality is assigned *a priori*, rather than having the status of a hypothesis to be verified. It is, in various ways, constitutive of the crime problem or, more accurately, the latter tends to be constructed as a question of criminal justice. In critical criminology and abolitionism the theme of social control developed by the Anglo-American sociology of deviance and control is assumed within a theoretical model, where social control is assimilated to domination, and domination, in turn, comes to acquire the traditional European connotations of negation, prohibition and repression. In this conception prison and the criminal justice system are central, representing the most clear and evident manifestation of the repressive power of the state and/or the dominant classes. It is on this basis that the entire theme of control is constructed. The relation between the criminal justice system and other agencies to which the production of social control may be imputed is then either ignored, or seen from the standpoint of the prison. The issue of crime thus becomes that of criminal justice, and from a perspective that enlarges the weight and significance of the latter (see chapter 1).

As far as the two types of realism are concerned, the problem of crime is constituted, albeit in opposite ways, by the definitions and practices deployed by the criminal justice system, thereby regaining a 'natural' status. It can in effect be said that in all these approaches, the sociological definition of crime coincides with that of the criminal justice system. For critical criminology and abolitionism what is criminal is what the criminal justice system defines as such; for the two realisms that which the criminal justice system defines as criminal is what is in truth 'criminal' – or universally perceived as harmful and to be condemned.

This coincidence carries simultaneous reductionist and distorting effects. If it is methodologically and theoretically reductionist to confine the issue of crime within the boundaries set by the criminal justice system, it is likewise a distortion to see the criminal justice system from the broad perspective of the criminal question. It would seem – and this is argued at greater length below – more productive to see the criminal question as constituted by a diversity of processes, not all reducible to the workings of the criminal justice system and whose, often conflictual, interaction can be taken into consideration only if their diversity is taken into account and if the centrality of the criminal justice system assumes the status of a hypothesis rather than remaining an unexamined presupposition.

In this chapter I set out to do two things. Firstly, I briefly outlined the centrality of 'responsibility' in its various senses both for the social sciences and common sense understandings of the relationships among human beings and between human beings and the world. While in the recent past explicit questions of responsibility had remained submerged, they have today powerfully resurfaced and are a dominant theme of public and political discourses. Within the social sciences, this takes the form of a new questioning of the problem of the actor. Secondly, I used 'responsibility' as a lens to read recent and contemporary approaches to the issues of crime and social control.

Before I follow up on these questions, and attempt to outline my own approach to them, I shall make a brief detour into the recent history of Italian 'criminologies'. This is necessary as this history is clearly different from those of British and American criminologies, though it appears to converge with them at the point when a 'critical criminology' emerged. In fact, this history may be of more general interest, precisely because such convergence, from so different a point of departure, could shed new light on the problems and paradoxes encountered by 'critical criminologies'.

3 Radical enquiries, unfounded policies

CONFUSION REIGNS: THE STATE OF ITALIAN CRIMINOLOGY

The importation of sociological treatments of deviance and social control is a recent phenomenon in Italy and comes up against two well-established traditions: jurisprudence and clinical criminology. If the object of study of the former is more the system of criminal law and procedure than the criminal justice system,[1] the object of the latter is the 'criminal'. Italian criminology is rather in fact forensic psychiatry, or investigation aimed at the reconstruction of the psychological dynamics of the individual offender (that is, obviously, individuals who have been arrested, tried and sentenced). I am aware that this excessive simplification does not do justice to criminological studies in Italy. It is indeed true that, within its specific orientations, Italian criminology has also, in recent years, taken account of tendencies in the criminology of other countries largely of a sociological orientation (see for example the last fifteen years of the journal *Rassegna di Criminologia*). Let us then say that sociological, clinical and psychiatric approaches have co-existed with alternating results, in a situation, however, characterised by the preponderant medical mould of Italian criminologists. This sustains a taken-for-granted attention to the single individual, seen as the 'end product' of processes and conditions which can indeed be 'social' but the reference to which is of interest predominantly in order to 'explain' or situate the behaviour of the single individual.

Rather than attempt a reconstruction of Italian criminology (see Faccioli 1984) I would like to limit myself to that sector, powerful academically and influential among practitioners in the criminal justice system, where criminology is directly engaged in practice: namely forensic psychiatry. In addition of course it is here that questions relating to responsibility cannot avoid being raised.

Traditionally in an ancillary position with respect to penal law, forensic psychiatry in Italy has been entrusted with the task of establishing scientifically the capacity of the accused to act from intention and will and, in the case of insanity, of possible social dangerousness. Such an institutional mandate is not without influence on the construction of the proper object of inquiry and the perception of the proper role of the criminologist. The couplet 'mental illness – social dangerousness' identifies two distinct tasks for the forensic psychiatrist, two different 'loyalties', the interweaving of two sets of professional standards. The professional standards of psychiatry, to which the forensic psychiatrist must turn when diagnosing insanity, call for an orientation to care, implying a priority to the defence of the interests of the sick. But as *forensic* psychiatrist, s/he has the duty of collaboration with the criminal justice system in the defence of the collective interest. Defence of the interests of the individual accused of criminal offending and orientation to social defence imply two different responsibilities, not infrequently contradictory and perceived as all the more so today, in the new scenario characterised by innovations in psychiatry and certain tendencies in criminal jurisprudence. We shall confront this theme in more detail in a subsequent chapter. Here my interest is to note how the present crisis of forensic psychiatry leads to attempts to redefine its own role drawing also on models influenced by the sociological criminologies currently on the market. To these I will refer therefore with a brief and selective picture of the Italian scene.

A 'new' criminology, distancing itself from the clinical and forensic psychiatric traditions began to assert itself in Italy during the early 1970s (see however Faccioli 1984 for a reconstruction which retraces the origins of this criminology in particular aspects of sociological interests as long ago as the beginning of the 1950s). It developed from an encounter between lawyers, workers in the criminal justice system, and sociologists who saw in the labelling paradigm a conceptual key to the workings of criminal justice in the context of a political programme for institutional reform and social change (Pitch 1982, introduction). Central to this encounter and to successive developments in the analysis of the issue of crime was the contribution of lawyers. This was a peculiarity of the Italian situation along with the already noted peculiarity of the strong academic base and influence of clinical criminology on criminal justice practitioners. It is therefore useful to underline briefly some aspects of the cultural environ- ment of jurisprudence during the period with which we are concerned.

Towards the end of the 1960s it is possible to identify the broad diffusion of two anti-formalist tendencies in the approach to law. A so-called 'strong' anti-formalism based on the revival of Marxian themes, in a form derived from the Frankfurt School, in which law and especially criminal law, was understood as a vehicle for the maintenance and reproduction of unjust social relations to be analysed by means of a demystifying critique. A 'weak' version of anti-formalism saw instead the question of law and criminal justice as a problem of the 'inadequacy' and excessive rigidity of legal procedures combined with the backwardness of the culture of judges in the face of social changes. Here the central theme was that of the proper implementation of the Italian Constitution. The first tendency took the form of the *critique of criminal law*, the second of the *critique of juridical culture*.

These anti-formalist tendencies emerged both in jurisprudence and among criminal justice professionals, and they interacted to create a climate favourable to the development of a theory of law and the judicial system which focused on their practical functioning rather than their normative aspects.[2] During the 1970s criminal law and the criminal justice system became central themes in the wider cultural and political debate: protagonists in the handling of social and political conflicts which simultaneously weakened their legitimacy and pushed them into the centre of the political arena.

The strong version of anti-formalism allied itself with anti-institutional and anti-authoritarian cultural currents and developed an analysis of the criminal justice system from the perspective of a critical demystification. There are three aspects of this form of analysis that are worth underlining: the centrality of the prison, both as a specific institution and even more as the symbol of the reproduction of domination; the elaboration of 'social control' as an aggregation of processes maintaining and reproducing domination; and the construction of the criminal question as an institutional question. The adoption of the labelling model within a Marxist paradigm meant that this criminology, in order to be critical, became a sociology of criminal law, focusing predominantly on the institutional side of the social reaction to 'crime'.[3] I am going to discuss this model further because it is by starting out from its aporias that I intend to confront the problem of how to study, today, the criminal question.

The anti-aetiological option – that it is not relevant to identify the causes of crime, but to analyse how crime is constructed by the processes of social control – denaturalises the notion of crime and, in principle, recognises its complex nature. However, the inclusion of this option within a Marxist paradigm produces some paradoxes. First of all, it tends to leave unexplored the processes through which certain phenomena and problems are selected as appropriate for the criminal justice system. These selection processes are taken as given by a form of analysis which understands institutions abstractly, photographically, separated from interaction with their subjects/objects. These latter in turn are understood in the same fixed, abstract way. The screening out of such processes results in a model which uncritically presupposes two distinct chains of causality: the first concerned with the origins of the phenomena, of the 'objective' social facts; the other with the formation of those processes and institutions which select from among the 'facts' and construct the *problems*. The relationship which is hypothesised between these two series of causes is circular and tautological. It is within this vicious circle that an anti-aetiological option is then affirmed. The status of cause is not problematised, neither is there any questioning of the consequences of operating within an epistemological framework which identifies two separate series of objects, causes and effects, where the one logically precedes and explains the other. In this scenario, then, the severance of the process of selection from interaction with the object of that selection, combined with the taking for granted of the basis of causality leads inevitably to functionalist interpretations. The 'causal' framework is taken for granted and confers meaning to an analysis in terms of functions.

In Italy, where within such a scenario the criminal justice system was the privileged focus, sophisticated interpretations of the logic of its functioning and legitimation have been produced, but to the neglect of issues concerning its formation and interaction with its subjects/objects. However, these interpretations did expose the genetic contradictions of the modern criminal justice system and the tensions to which it is continually exposed.[4]

Another fundamental issue which this model takes as resolved is that of the theoretical status of the concept of social problem. Here the interrelation between theoretical hypotheses and criminal and social policy orientations was crucial. The model theorises social problems as complex constructions, results of the interaction between 'real' needs, the perceptions of these needs given within a particular historical situation, and the selective processes of the agencies of social control. The point is that this model provides an implicit solution to the question of the 'reality' of needs, situating it within the 'material contradictions of capitalist society'. This has resulted in the lack of a critical perspective on the ways in which social questions and their meanings are formed, tending rather to deduce them entirely from (and as the inverse of) institutional responses. The latter, in their turn, are derived from the 'requirements of capitalism'. 'Real' needs are thus defined as that which the institutional responses are repressing, eluding and negating. Again, a vicious circularity both enabled and concealed, by choosing as interlocutors actors – institutional and social – who perceived themselves as participants in a single and unitary political project. Take the example of crimes against property, which tend to be emphasised in a 'Marxist' perspective. By starting from the dynamics of selection by the agencies of social control, it seemed easy to make the leap on one hand to 'unemployment' or 'marginalisation', and on the other to 'defence of class interests' and to the issue of the reproduction of the social relations of production (including the reproduction of criminality itself); from here one was able to make a further leap to the suggestion of policies aimed both at the radical restructuring of social relations, and the reform of the criminal justice system. That it was a question of leaps rather than of a necessary and inevitable journey, remained hidden thanks to a particular – and brief – political conjuncture. Successive events have demonstrated that the 'reality' of needs cannot be consigned to the metaphysics of 'the contradictions of capitalist society', nor deduced from institutional responses, and not even left to the formulations of those who are regarded as the bearers of these needs. Rather, these three dimensions are not commensurable, they are not part of the same political project.

The present crisis of this model is the result of the more general theoretical and political crisis of Marxist paradigms. For the study of the criminal question, the disappearance of an interlocutor (real or imaginary) to whom to address a politics of crime, puts into context the problem of the 'foundations' of the politics of reform. Of this more later.

In Italy, the decline of the radical project, the fragmentation of totalizing models of the social has led the left in the sociology of criminal law and criminology to a critical pessimism which, while not rejecting politics, prefers to concentrate on the defence and revitalisation of the very legal safeguards and procedures which were neglected by the analysis predominant in the previous period but which have been threatened in recent years by so-called emergency legislation and judicial practices. (See among others, Baratta, Silbernagl 1983; Bricola 1982; the debates in AA.VV. 1977; AA.VV. 1979; Ferrajoli 1977; 1984).[5]

The question of (civil) rights acquires a centrality itself symptomatic of the revival of the 'problem of the actor'. We will examine its consequences in later chapters in the context of the debates on juvenile justice, on the relation between psychiatry and criminal justice and on the symbolic use of penal justice on the part of collective actors. On the theoretical level, however, the tendency to remain within the perimeters defined by the criminal justice system[6] risks leading to an invocation of rights based on abstract appeals to principle. If the connections between policies and institutions of criminal justice on the one hand and social policies and institutions on the other, is not grasped, the question of the relationship or contradiction between civil rights and social rights can be lost. The result is a return to a purely defensive formalism, of little use on the theoretical level and politically evasive (for an analysis that avoids this difficulty see Marconi 1983a).

The centrality of the criminal justice system remains however, both in clinical and critical criminology and in the sociology of criminal law. In the present scenario clinical criminologists are led to a questioning of the status of actor of the 'criminal', of the 'degrees of freedom' which it is possible to attribute to him/her and on one's own professional competences regarding such issues. This takes place in the framework of legislative innovations, such as the new Italian code of penal procedure and the so-called Gozzini law on penal reform and the discussion regarding the possibility of introducing, alongside the expert opinion of the psychiatrist, that of the criminologist. Such innovations introduce flexibility and differentiation in the sentencing process, widening the margins of judicial discretion and therefore opening up a wider field of 'expert' competence. (Succeeding chapters will return at length to this point.)

Sociologists and lawyers on the 'left' are instead involved in a questioning of the status of the rights of liberty in the context of the welfare state. As has been noted, the underlying question concerns the emergence of the more general issue of the status of the individual actor: an issue which however cannot be confronted within the traditional confines of the debate on crime.

I shall now return to a discussion of my approach to the issues of crime and social control.

HOW TO STUDY THE CRIMINAL QUESTION

Defining the criminal question

To study the criminal question is different from studying crime. It means that crime is not considered independently from the procedures by which it is defined, the instruments deployed in its administration and control and the politics and debate around criminal justice and public order. The criminal question can therefore be provisionally defined as an area constituted by actions, institutions, policies and discourses whose boundaries shift. If the reference to criminal justice as the place where actions become defined as crimes is fundamental, nevertheless to reduce the criminal question to a question of criminal justice leads to a failure to explore the latter, to confer on it a sort of fixity and rigidity impermeable to relations with other institutions. It leads, furthermore, to a formalism which, while perhaps useful for contrasting substantialist and correctional theories, models and political positions, reveals a sterility in its inability to grasp just what makes the criminal question a complex question: the interconnections between social questions, institutional responses, conflicts and policies in which criminal law, besides providing a language and terminology, plays within many different games.

An old, though anything but out of date or faded, dispute counterposes those who consider crime as that and only that which is so defined by criminal law at a given moment to those who either hypostatise existing criminal law as the expression of some type of meta-historical general will, or postulate it as the embodiment of a set of 'natural' interests or needs, and understand by criminality the violation of norms which have a deeper foundation from which criminal law is (or ought to be) legitimated.[7] The first tendency risks neglecting the significance which 'crime' socially and culturally assumes in an often conflictual relationship with criminal justice and penal policies. The second tendency annuls the tension between juridical norms and social and cultural norms, and while it deduces its object from criminal law, it in fact excludes criminal law itself from inspection.

The problem, among sociologists, has generally been seen as that of the autonomy of academic disciplines: of whether it is satisfactory to borrow the definitions of the object of study from outside, from law, or whether it is possible, necessary and legitimate to construct it autonomously. Does taking the definition of criminality from law mean assuming law's reasoning, embracing its political assumptions? How much real autonomy do or can 'sociological' definitions of crime have? This problem has been in part avoided by making crime a subcategory of 'deviance', the latter being defined autonomously (at least in appearance). However that was simply a way of displacing the problem (on the debates on the definition of deviance see Pitch 1982). Among sociologists and criminologists therefore, the dispute between formalism and substantialism (in law) became that of dependence versus independence of sociological formulations from those of law, a question with explicit political aspects and which has often been confronted in terms of the role and function of the criminologist.[8]

A decisive turn with the labelling theorists, was the choice as a proper object of analysis – or as a way of identifying deviance and criminality – of that which is identified as such by the processes of 'social reaction'. In other words, law and criminal justice institutions are not only seen as constituting the category of crime, but, at least in principle, are seen as interacting with other processes of social reaction. This type of argument moves away from formalism (though it can become wholly formalist) to a constructionist perspective. It becomes possible to speak of the 'criminal question' rather than of 'criminality'. The object of analysis is no longer 'borrowed from law', neither is it defined in terms of an impossible autonomy from law. Questions of dependence or independence – and the associated political implications – emerge in a quite different way.

The adoption of a constructionist perspective has both de-naturalised and de-formalised the conception of crime. To construct one's object of study in terms of the criminal question does not imply at all the denial of the 'real' existence of single acts or complexes of actions which have negative consequences for the lives, interests, values of individuals or social groups. It means nevertheless to examine how, why and with what consequences these acts or complexes of acts come to be confronted as crimes. It implies the possibility and the necessity of taking into account – without absolutising them – different points of view, including of course one's own, and to be aware of the fact that the sociologist and the criminologist themselves contribute to the construction of the criminal question through their analyses, discourses, political interventions and debates.

The constructionist perspective likewise allows us to see the obvious: that the term 'crime' refers to a completely incoherent variety of acts and behaviours which have in common only that they are regarded as crimes. What relationship can possibly be identified between the violation of obscure administrative norms, robbery with violence, and, let us say, the export of capital in violation of currency rules? It therefore allows us to ask why these acts are seen as crimes, and other acts, perceived by some groups or individuals as similarly or more seriously injurious to their interests are not.

What 'the public' think of as crime and what, according to 'the public' should be considered crime, or what cultural and symbolic significance is carried by law and criminal justice, is an integral aspect of the criminal question.

To refrain from either assuming the centrality of criminal justice or isolating it as a standpoint does not mean, however, proposing a mode of analysis – a construction of the object of study, the development of models, categories and instruments – which is all inclusive, totalizing, or worse, *ad hoc*: a 'science' of the criminal question. That would be equivalent to a reification identical to that deployed by criminologies (both traditional and otherwise) and fall foul of the tautology and circularity of such approaches. The criminal question, naturally, exists only in the sense of indicating a particular nexus of problems and/or a particular visual angle from which to look at other problems.

Causes and politics

Any project of intervention in the criminal question, or particular aspects of it, implies, as has been noted, a certain, more or less explicit and formalised, idea of the 'causes' of such questions. Rather, the way the problem is posed and defined implies a strategy for its solution which in turn presupposes specific causes.

The paradigm problem–solution presupposes a research programme in which the first move, temporally and logically, is the investigation of the nature of the problem followed by intervention (for a discussion of this paradigm in the area of psychiatry and justice, see De Leonardis 1988). In this programme the problem is given, it is clearly independent of the way in which the researcher formulates it, and its nature becomes understood through the discovery of its causes. The truth of the problem, that which is given by its causes, is a guarantee that the solution proposed is the correct one. This paradigm, as has already been said, forms the predominant basis of progressive policies. As far as 'crime' is concerned, the attempts to force it into the strait-jacket of this model have given rise to a variety of 'aetiological' criminologies and sociologies of which we have taken note. Approaches which reject this orientation are frequently denounced as decisionist, conservative, formalist and politically abstentionist. They may certainly be read as uninterested in understanding if by the latter is meant 'discovery of causes', and driven only by explicitly 'political' objectives, where politics is conceived as that decision which is concerned with the solution of problems.

We face, then, two approaches at first sight diametrically opposed: on one side the argument that the causal understanding of a problem is indispensable to (and therefore precedes) its resolution, on the other the affirmation that problem and solution are relatively autonomous, and that the solution necessarily corresponds to the functional requisites of the system in which it emerges rather than to the causes of the problem. The reference here is to Luhmann and his school more than to the administrative and managerial criminologists which were noted above. To deny the validity of a causal understanding follows from a strategy of intervention aimed not at 'resolving' the problem, but rather at the preservation and reproduction of the (juridical, political etc.) subsystems involved.

The identification of understanding with the discovery of (ultimate, true) causes is linked to a conception of politics as a form of intervention whose objectives are *founded* on a scientifically attainable truth from which they derive rationality and necessity. The politics of the left, inspired by Marxism, has also often been formulated in this way. The supremacy of the plan, though on one side appearing as the supremacy of politics and conscious decision making, in reality draws its legitimacy and strength from the notion of its foundation on a scientific analysis of reality from which its objectives inexorably flow. This results in a circularity which paradoxically excludes the dimensions of choice and preference. The relation between theory and practice may be, and has often been, formulated in a completely opposite manner: but until this relation is inscribed in a teleologically oriented model, in which history has *one* sense and *one* direction, the results cannot but be those I described.

The paradigm problem–solution cannot take account of unintended consequences: they are at the most errors, attributable to an incorrect application of the theoretical model or to a lack of political will, or to ignorance, disinterest, and bad faith of those charged with implementation of the policies.

Is it possible to understand without going in search of causes? Can non-'founded' objectives be posed? The choice of objectives involves a decision which cannot be founded on the transparency of an absolute rationality. Such decisions govern the understanding of the problem, in the sense that the latter comes to be posed in terms of this decision. But the decision on the choice of objectives, in its turn, can only be provisional, subjected to modifications as the problem changes under the pressure of its solution. This is a strategy of research and intervention which does not force reality into the strait-jacket of objectives given *a priori* and which sees understanding as an interactive process between different actors, including, obviously, the sociologist herself.

A 'criminology' which is non-aetiological is not thereby necessarily pessimistic, abstentionist, or one which does not take positions. On the contrary, it can be the programme of participant observers[9] aware that their analyses of the problem, inspired by, rather than logically derived from their own choices and preferences, enters into the formation of the problem itself. Problems and solutions are not separable, neither are they given once and for all. The 'unintended' consequences of solutions are not necessarily errors or deviations: they allude rather to the limits of politics as a rational project and to the limits of a theoretical paradigm which adopts linear models of cause and effect.

A problem of standpoint

The following appeared in the *Wall Street Journal* (28 June 1988):

> Frontier justice. The return of vigilantism in America carries a clear lesson: the system of criminal justice constructed by liberals over the last 20 years to protect Americans has failed the task of protecting the people who most have need of it.

So now people are providing their own defence. This trend is less evident in Italy, but even here research (see Olgiati, Astori 1988) indicates the proliferation, if not of vigilantes, of private police. The two phenomena are different – the first relates, at least in the light of the examples reported in the American newspaper, to attempts at defence undertaken within under-privileged groups and strata towards activity within these groups themselves: it speaks of the spread of a rising sense of insecurity, above all in the metropolitan centres, accompanied by a lack of confidence in the institutional agencies of social control. The second refers rather to a multiplication and diversification of goods and interests such that their protection by public agencies no longer appears sufficient. This implies, further, that the identification of injury to these goods and interests as crimes is becoming of less concern than preventing such injury occurring in the first place (on the low productivity of the criminal justice system see Marconi 1984). Additionally it implies that these goods and interests are not or are not perceived of, as common, collective, universalisable. There is also another phenomenon connected to this, namely, the spread, above all in large private organisations, of autonomous systems of control and punishment for transgressions, not only of specific organisational norms but also of norms liable to sanction by criminal law (Spector 1981). Acts which would be recognised as crimes are dealt with by systems of internal justice, inflicting private sanctions.

These three phenomena can be analysed in different ways. I have introduced them here only to underline a theme already mentioned several times: the unstable and irregular boundaries of the criminal question and the necessity therefore always to understand it as the provisional result of processes which have their origins in, and are acted out by, different actors.[10]

Does the growth of vigilantism in the black and Hispanic ghettos of large American cities speak really, or only, of the failure of 'liberal' criminal justice policies? Such a formulation is interesting in that it seems to underplay the 'causes' of violence and crime in these deprived areas, but, critical of liberal policies, attacks both a 'solution' and a particular way of looking at the 'problem'. It sees policies based on the idea that 'criminality' has roots in marginality, unemployment, discrimination, and that the 'criminals' are themselves also victims to be rehabilitated and re-educated, as policies which harm the very social strata for whom they were devised to protect. Such is demonstrated by the fact that members of these groups are organising themselves for self-defence, outside the law, often using violence and thereby committing in their turn further 'crimes'. This argument can be located in the repertoire of conservative 'realism', but that is of less interest here, than the fact that it simplifies a complex situation.

Two further explanations, likewise oversimplified, could be offered. According to the first, let us call it the classical liberal one, vigilantism is caused not by the failure of liberal policies but by their incorrect implementation: crime and violence are caused by marginalisation and poverty and as long as these latter are not eradicated the former will grow and produce similarly violent reactions in the populations victimised by them. According to the second, let us call it critical, interpretation, vigilantism has to be understood rather as a war amongst the poor: 'criminality' and violence are indicators of objective social problems, but the way in which they are perceived and handled by the poor themselves is the result of policies only partially to be seen as failures. In reality such policies can be said to succeed to the extent that they have imposed their definitions of the problem (criminality rather than oppression or exploitation). Vigilantism is therefore a symptom of profound neglect and of . . . false consciousness.

None of these three formulations leaves the classical perimeters of the criminal question. In each one of course there are some sensible observations, insights which can be shared to the extent that they do not claim to grasp the totality of the question but only reflect on partial aspects of it. The identification of an aspect as specific and partial, analysable with specific categories and instruments, adequate to that aspect, has the highest probability of grasping the connections and the relations with other aspects than does the application of a model where the connections are already implicit, given by the model itself, and therefore where the object of analysis is constructed as unitary, entirely derived from a viewpoint taken as privileged. It does not matter how complicated are the interconnections provided for in the model: the object so constructed is diluted and simplified.

In the case under discussion, for example, the question is not so much, or only, that multiple and different explanations can exist of the emergence of this type of vigilantism, as that this phenomenon can be examined from many points of view: its implications concerning the capacity for self-organisation, the level of available economic cultural and social resources, the dynamic of relations between citizens and institutions, what conceptions of 'justice' enter into play, etc. Each of these questions, and others that can be formulated, allude to areas traditionally separated (in terms of academic disciplines) each of which offers a specific conceptual and methodological set of instruments, not containable within the classical perimeters of the criminal question and its *ad hoc* formulations in criminology and sociology.

An analogous discourse can be developed around the proliferation of private policing or the diffusion of autonomous systems of justice in large corporations. There is a certain theme, however, in all three examples, which seems to me inescapable: that of the criminal question as a starting point for processes and systems of control in conflict and interaction among themselves.

The vigilantism mentioned by the *Wall Street Journal* is not only an indicator – and certainly not, in my opinion, the main one – of a resurgence of acts of crime and violence in the metropolitan ghettos, it is also an example of 'informal justice', born out of fragmented social relations – nothing to do with the 'community' of the abolitionists – and which expresses itself in a more ferocious way than institutional justice. It indicates also, therefore, an emergence of extreme forms of social control which have to be understood in relation not only to the supposed failure or insufficiency of the processes of control by the criminal justice system, but also to the crisis, insufficiency and loss of legitimacy of those processes of control inherent in the work of service agencies, both public and private, from the school to the various agencies of social work.[11] What is involved is the very structure of relations between individuals, groups and institutions.

As far as the proliferation of private policing is concerned, it seems that this is a phenomenon both equal and opposite to that of the vigilantism of the ghetto. Whereas vigilantism takes on the defence, no matter how inappropriate and inadequate, of conditions of life increasingly deteriorating and seen as threatened, private policing signifies the multiplication of autonomous forms of protection on the part of groups, organisations, and individuals which are economically and socially powerful. It alludes to the diffusion of apparatuses paralleling those of the state, with the difference that the first are unhindered by bureaucratic slowness, lack of resources, and legal constraints. Private police forces do not defend 'the community' but the goods and the interests of those who employ them. This poses at least two questions: one concerning the efficiency, legitimation and functions of the criminal justice system; the other concerning the ambiguous duplication of some of these functions through their privatisation.[12] Such developments are helping to change, in ways still hardly understood, the meaning and content of 'crime', and also most likely, what is meant by justice.

Similar questions are raised by the systems of private sanctions administered by large organisations which identify and handle both transgressions of no criminal relevance, and those which would become crimes if they came to the knowledge of the public authorities. The results of these systems of sanctions interact with those produced by the systems of public control.

In a society like ours the systems and processes of control are many: what emerges as crime is the residual product of their, often conflictual, interaction. The criminal question must then be conceived not so much, or not only, as a specific object of analysis but as a problematic site from which to observe this interaction.

Questions of responsibility

As we have seen, questions of responsibility are by no means exhausted in the (fictitious) contrast between the responsibility of the authors of criminal acts and the responsibility of society for them and towards them. This way of putting the question, however, makes explicit what the dominating sociologies and criminologies of the past thirty years implied. Their being interpreted in deterministic terms was facilitated by their aetiological programme, but, though permitted by those same sociologies, it was a distorted interpretation. Such interpretation was due to the eclipse of the social actor in paradigms which variously combined the search of linear causal links with functionalist models.[13]

The relations between social science and criminal law have been the object of a vast literature, which I am not going to review here.[14] These relations have been seen as a conflict between two opposed, yet interacting, conceptions of truth and methodologies for obtaining it. On the one hand the empirical 'truth' arrived at by the inductive methods of social science, and on the other the processual 'truth', arrived at through deduction from legal principles. To each of these methodologies would appear to correspond strategies of intervention also necessarily opposed to each other. On the one hand 'expert' intervention on criminogenic social conditions, ranging from social engineering to rehabilitation and care, informed by social science and seen as manipulatory or emancipatory, according to ideological standpoint. On the other, the defence of individual rights and basic liberties through (criminal) law. The objectives of these strategies would appear to correspond to two different models of social control. The one, non-repressive, oriented to persuasion to conformity, pervasive and totalizing, informed by the social sciences; the other oriented to dissuade from transgression, purely retributive, corresponding to law. Where the first model could seem to dispense with ascribing consciousness and intentionality to the object of its intervention, the second functions precisely on the basis of such ascription.

If the system of criminal justice[15] shows itself in reality to operate by means of correctionist models variously inscribed within a retributivist frame,[16] the processes of social control informed by and which in turn inform the various social sciences demonstrate a similar degree of dependence on mixed models, through which they produce, albeit in different ways, an ascription of consciousness and intentionality.

In other chapters we will confront in more detail the current forms taken by the relation between criminal justice, with its legal discourses, and agencies for treatment and assistance, with their accompanying psychiatric, psychological and sociological knowledges. We shall look at this issue in the areas of juvenile justice and the criminal responsibility of the mentally ill. What I would like to bring out here is that the tension between 'treatment' and punishment is as much to do with the criminal justice system as it is with the systems of welfare and social services.[17]

The notion of desert is linked both to retributive and distributive justice. Not only is the distribution of resources and services regulated – even in universalist oriented welfare systems – on the basis of degrees of responsibility of the client for the conditions which result in resources and services being requested: the actual dispensing of resources depends on decisions of the professional in evaluating the 'desert' of the user her/himself (Reamer 1982).[18] It is certainly necessary to distinguish between services intended for all, based on the recognition of universal social rights such as health, and forms of particular assistance based on the existence or recognition of specific situations. It is in this second case that the judgement of desert is predominantly visible. The more the social worker is convinced of the 'innocence' of the client – of the fact of her not being blameworthy for her unfortunate circumstances, the more probable is it that assistance will be forthcoming.

Historically, however, the welfare model as such is constructed precisely on the presumption of innocence of the victims, or in other words on the basis of a determinism which tends to exclude the conscious participation of the victims themselves in the creation of their misfortune. The fact that present social policies are not immune from considerations of this type is demonstrated by the debates, particularly sharp in a period of crisis of the welfare state, on the boundaries of collective responsibility, the criteria for access to services, and on what ought to be and what can be considered as social rights.

In reality the work of the social services seems to operate prevalently (Reamer 1982) with a model of 'soft' determinism in which the assumption of the free will of the user coexists with that of his being constrained by circumstances beyond his control. This makes possible oscillating attitudes on the part of the professionals, and a distribution of services differentiated on the basis of the status of the client, even when such distribution is seen as a right. It is not only a question of the quality of resources distributed which is at issue here, but also the type of resources and the forms of distribution. The presumption of the innocence of the client involves the latter handing over to the professional the decisions concerning the solutions to the problems for which intervention was requested.

The tension between care and punishment is revealed in models of welfare which oscillate between the two paradigms. Historically, the emphasis on the innocence of the client has been a characteristic of social democratic policies, while the emphasis on the responsibility of the client was emphasised by conservative policies.

The question presents itself today in a different way (see De Leonardis 1988a). The inclusive logic of the welfare state has enlarged the sphere of substantive, social rights. The distribution of services and resources is based decreasingly on the identification of special areas of need, and increasingly on the recognition of the right to welfare of all citizens independently of their social and economic characteristics, labour market position, etc. That has involved the growth of a new contractual capacity of citizens towards the institutions, and a new conception of the responsibility of the institutions towards them. The tension between a handing over by clients of responsibility for resolving their problems to the social service agencies and the blaming of the client by the agencies (in the form of denial of resources, neglect, delegation to separate custodial and correctional institutions) has tended to transform itself into a new tension between rights to liberty and social rights of the citizen/client. The growth of movements and single issue groups such as committees for rights of the sick, associations of families of drug dependants and mentally ill etc., both reflects and pushes forward this transformation. The issue of responsibility becomes articulated and enriched, it becomes the focus of conflict and interaction between citizens and institutions and of the debate within the institutions themselves.

Indeed, cure and care by welfare institutions, insofar as they are rights, imply a double obligation on the part of the professionals: these rights impose on them the obligation to cure and care for and at the same time to respect the eventual will of the client, who remains a full-fledged citizen, to refuse such cure and care.[19] Here there is the potential for a concept of professional responsibility which does not negate, but on the contrary emphasises, interacts with and constructs the responsibility of the client: and vice versa. Responsibility becomes, and it becomes possible to conceive it as, not a property which is intrinsic to the conscious actor by definition, but a product of the interaction through which, reciprocally, we construct ourselves as actors.

Constraints and responsibility

If Davis (1983) is right, that 'what distinguishes criminal law from other means of social control (treatment, terror, conditioning etc.) is that it presupposes individuals who (a) can follow rules or not, according to choice (b) can be persuaded to follow rules by the distant prospect of an established penalty' – in other words the presupposition of rationality defined as the possibility of adapting one's actions in the light of circumstances distant and uncertain – then it has to be admitted that this distinction performs a purely symbolic function as long as the concrete practice of the criminal justice system is articulated rather through 'treatment, terror, conditioning'. Neither do the other forms of social control, nowadays at least, escape the tensions of the recognition of rationality.

There is nevertheless, a difference: in criminal law the rationality of the agent is presupposed, in the 'other means of social control' it may be constructed. In both it is the object of conflict. In both, responsibility is understood as predicated on freedom of choice under conditions of constraint: there is no freedom without the establishment of rules (see the apt comments of Walzer on the Biblical text of Exodus, Walzer 1985). The counterposing of criminal law with 'other means of social control' refers to a juxtaposition of different types of constraints. The constraints of law are explicit, the result of political decisions understandable as the result of a 'social contract' or as imposed by a dominant group, devised to protect goods and interests which are thereby constituted as collective and universal, sanctioned by penalties established in advance. The second refers to implicit limits to action, conditions of action specific to each actor and each situation, resulting from the history of that particular actor. Such a contrast has often been made to correspond to that between action and behaviour: the first as based on ends and norms, the second reducible to determining causes. Criminal law would then have to be concerned with intentional action, other means of social control with determined behaviour. The former would reconfirm tautologically a presupposed responsibility, the latter would confirm an absence of responsibility likewise presupposed.

It has already been explained how this distinction is fictitious, and how the question of responsibility tends to present itself today in a new way even within the 'other means of social control'. This implies problems and contradictions for criminal law and the criminal justice system which will be examined later. But it is the question of the nature of the constraints, and therefore of the way of understanding rationality and social action which is more generally at issue.

The present philosophical and sociological debate on social action, the status of the actor, the types of rationality is very rich and articulated, and goes well beyond the limited scope of this book (see among others, Boudon 1980; Giddens 1987, chaps. 1, 3 and 4; Elster 1978, 1983; Ricoeur 1986; for an Italian discussion: Balbo *et al.* 1985; De Leonardis 1987; Donolo, Fichera 1988). I only want to reflect on how the question of the responsibility of the actor may be posed in relation to, on one side 'constraints', on the other 'unintended consequences'. I am working within a conceptual framework in which the social actor is conceived as in a position to understand and will that which she does, to give explanations for her actions in terms of motivations and intentions (see the distinction in Ricoeur 1986, especially chaps 2 and 4) and where, above all, these explanations – the self-accounts of the actors – are held to be a constitutive aspect of the action itself. This does not mean however, (a) that everything the actors know is contained in and therefore extractable from that which they are able to say that they know. There is, in fact, a shared knowledge of procedures and practices which is unconscious in the sense of being taken for granted. The typical example is that of speaking a language. In speaking we utilise a complex and sophisticated knowledge of grammatical and lexical rules and syntax etc. which we are not in a position, if asked, to elaborate or describe. This shared knowledge constructs the context of social life; (b) that social action is not 'free' and that it is not 'determined'. In its existence, within the routines of daily life, it is both 'limited' by the shared knowledge and contributes to producing (and reproducing) it. Constraints are not causes: rather they are products and conditions of action; (c) that not all the consequences of action are 'willed': which does not mean that the actors are impelled by causes which determine the course of their actions beyond what is contained in their intentions. Unintended consequences can arise as the result of more complex interactions (see Boudon 1980) both in the short run (as in the example of a bank failure as the consequence of a rush by individuals to withdraw their money when the word is spread of its insolvency: no one wants the bank to fail, each individual wants only to withdraw their own money), and the long term. Thus no one wants the planet to die from pollution, or closer to home the pollution of the Mediterranean. When we say that these are the results of a certain type of industrial and technological development we are saying that they are the unintended (nowadays increasingly less so!) results of collective and individual choices – seen in the recent period as less inevitable by virtue of becoming the object of increasingly sharp political conflicts.

The theme of unintended consequences throws new light on the relationship between constraints and intentional action. Elster (1983) shows how actors can pose constraints on their future action, on the basis of predictions of a future preference the consequences of which, at present, they judge harmful. The present 'I' constrains the future 'I' in order to protect itself against the risk of a preference that, at present, it considers harmful.[20] The imposition of constraints on the basis of our present choices implies that the present preferences are to be considered rational, the future ones potentially irrational, inadequate and dangerous. The position of juridical and social norms may also be read in these terms.[21]

In this case the consequences are expected and predicted. That implies, then, that it is necessary to reduce to the minimum the possibility of unintended, unpredicted consequences, such that the imposition of constraints will be rational, that is efficacious. The aim of knowledge is to control nature, society and oneself so as to protect oneself against the risk of consequences, at present, not desired. Ulysses must know both where the Sirens are and what effect their songs have on those who hear them, and also, what he himself, being human, will probably desire to do on hearing them. We can interpret the history of Western science, at least from the 17th century onwards, in this way.[22] The scientific prediction of the future, as with the choices we make in the present, is value laden and an object of conflict (see Douglas and Wildavsky 1983) – all the more so, as the instruments of knowledge at our disposal increase in sophistication (see Jonas 1984).

Naturally however, unintended consequences occur not only in the more distant future, but also in the short term, in the same arc of time in which our present action unfolds. A mixture of intended and unintended consequences of our preceding actions configure the constraints within which our present action moves: even those choices, policy decisions and legal norms oriented to placing explicit constraints on our future action. The question of responsibility poses itself therefore in a context of *constraints*, not of *causes*. From this some obvious considerations follow. The bringing into relationship of action and *unintended* consequences is always a process of revealing constraints. Conversely the bringing into the light of constraints can be seen as a process of enlarging the sphere of responsibility.

Turning back to the distinction between criminal law and 'other means of social control'. This distinction corresponds to that between criminality and illness, deprivation etc., i.e. between constraints explicitly imposed and voluntarily transgressed and implicit constraints, involuntarily transgressed. Which concrete actions fall into one or the other of these categories involves, as is well known, the interaction of many factors (the voluntary taking of modest quantities of psychotropic substances – what psychotropic substances are considered illegal at a particular time and which are not is a further point in this argument – was up until 1975, in Italy, a crime. Now it is an illness.[23]) We might though interrogate this distinction from another angle. The constraints constituted by juridical norms prefigure consequences, for the actor, if s/he violates them, which add themselves to the consequences of the action as such. If the latter can be unintended, the former, as a matter of principle, are foreseen and predictable. I do not wish anyone to be killed as a result of my driving the car too fast. I know however, or I ought to know, that if such occurs then I will incur punishment. The process of the attribution of responsibility which leads to punishment, however, implies precisely that it is to the former set of consequences that I must answer, i.e. that even these should have been predicted and expected by me: I *did not wish* to kill, but I should have been aware that it could have happened in consequence of my reckless driving. What I mean to say is that, if, as Davis (1983) points out, criminal law as a means of social control presupposes actors in a position to take account of the legal consequences of the violation of its norms – in other words, its effectiveness relies on threat and works through deterrence – criminal law also initiates a reverse process. The norm constitutes at the same time an area of non-juridical consequences which the actor should have predicted and to which the actor is expected to respond. The positing of legal norms extends the area of predictability and, in this sense, the range of consequences to which an actor can be called to answer, hence also the area of imputation of intentionality, of 'free choice'.

Sociological arguments for a minimalist criminal law

Emerging on one hand as a 'third position' between left realism and abolitionism, on the other as consistent with the development of a concern by the left with legal guarantees of due process in opposition to the law and order policies of the 'state of emergency' in Italy during the 1970s, the thesis of Minimalist criminal law characterises a good part of the sociology of criminal law, of critical criminology, and the philosophy of criminal law in Italy. (See the special issue of the journal *Dei Delitti e delle Pene*, 3, 1985). This position must be seen as a value option, as the choice of a criminal policy arising from judgements about the concrete functioning of the criminal justice system. Reductionist precedents in the sphere of punitive intervention by the state are also retraceable to classical liberal theories of crime and punishment, and a return to these principles is a fundamental part of the idea of minimal penal intervention.

Briefly, this idea developed in the context of the critical analysis of the criminal justice system referred to above. The main themes have been summarised (see Baratta 1985): punishment as 'institutional violence' or rather as a legal limitation of rights and needs; criminal justice as functioning in a selective manner, both as regards goods and interests which it protects, and as regards the process of criminalisation and the 'recruitment of its clients'. The system of punishment produces more problems than it claims to solve. Up to this point there is no difference between this analysis and that underlying abolitionist proposals. The political proposals are, however, profoundly different. While the policies of alternatives to, or progressive abolition of the prison as the main or virtually exclusive form of modern punishment are themes of discussion, not only in 'critical' circles but also in those of government and international organisations, proposals to abolish criminal law are contested (see Ferrajoli 1985, 1989) through a recourse to utilitarian justifications of punishment. In summary, according to Ferrajoli, it is not enough to justify punishment, which is itself an evil, in terms of the prevention of similar crimes on the part of the offender or others: this would take the form of a 'utilitarianism cut in half'. It is necessary instead to refer to an additional utilitarian parameter: 'the maximum possible good of the non-deviants, and the minimum harm to the deviants'. Punishment, according to Ferrajoli, has as its primary purpose the prevention of unjust infliction of pain: 'it does not protect only the person harmed by the crime, but also protects the offender from informal public or private reactions'. This perspective leaves no doubt that the criminal justice system actually functions in quite another way, or, conversely, that other systems than criminal justice would be more efficient if the sole purpose were that of preventing and repressing crime. But while such alternatives carry insupportably high costs in terms of civil liberties, it is precisely as a basis for a coherent critique of the criminal justice system and the present politics of crime control that this perspective is informative.

I would like to argue for this perspective in the politics of crime control from a different point of view. It is perhaps true today that the criminal law, with respect to other 'means of social control' at least offers major guarantees in principle respectful of the civil liberties of those who violate it. But it is not impossible to imagine the introduction of a system of such guarantees within a rethought and reconstructed 'other means of social control'[24] particularly if the latter were radically rethought and devised[25] explicitly as a means of social control (see Baratta 1985). Besides, there is the fact that criminal law can defend from unjust punishments if it is socially legitimated: and legitimation, despite what the supporters of an interpretation of legitimation in exclusively procedural terms say, appears to have much to do with efficacy.

However, according to my preceding discussion, the imposition of legal norms can be seen as one of the more simple ways, less subject to equivocation, of putting constraints on future actions: explicit, determinate constraints, susceptible to being annulled or modified, I do not say by rational consensus, but at least through conflicts which cannot avoid having or acquiring an immediate political significance. The historical and conventional status of such constraints is more evident than in other cases and therefore it is easier to argue their possible injustice, inefficiency or backwardness in particular cases.

Such constraints also, at least in principle, constitute precise areas of intended consequences[26] and thus by delimiting it, confer significance and content to individual liberty. In order for that to happen, it is necessary that the sphere of intervention of criminal justice be reduced as far as possible, the legal issues clearly identified, the punishments definite.

A politics of minimal legal intervention, however, cannot be considered in isolation from those types of social policy productive of other forms of constraints, in addition to their role in the delivery and distribution of resources, for all the reasons already elaborated above. But there is an ulterior motive here which it would be useful to study attentively. As will be better described in the next chapter, we are witnessing today an increase in the use of the symbolic potential of criminal justice. The process of 'new criminalisation' – the criminalisation of actions, events, questions hitherto not considered crimes – often initiated and encouraged by social movements, can be seen as an aspect of a tendency to reintroduce questions of personal responsibility. Here it can only be a matter however, of a responsibility which is constitutive of actors abstracted from any other constraint, mere bearers of 'negative' rights. A surely necessary fiction, but one which meets, on the side of the 'criminal' with the cumbersome presence of a personal history which cannot but make reference to other responsibilities: and on the part of those who have to occupy themselves in various ways with the 'criminal' (police, judges, prison officers, social workers, etc.) with the delicate and fragile equilibrium which would have to be maintained between the attribution of responsibility (to the criminal) and assumption of responsibility for the consequences relative to the decisions concerning the choice of interventions: questions which refer directly to bodies of knowledge and agencies of treatment and welfare and produce a different responsibility, more complex and articulate: a responsibility *for*.[27]

4   Rather riders than horses?

The use of the symbolic potential of criminal
justice by actors in conflict[1]

A generally neglected aspect of the question of crime concerns the
demands for criminalisation; the ways in which problems and social
conflicts become identified as appropriate subjects for criminal justice.
Today, however, this aspect is becoming increasingly important. Alongside
a certain loss of legitimacy of the criminal justice system (due to low
productivity, low efficiency, conflicts and changes within the judiciary, see
on this point Ferrarese 1984), there is a consistent, and in many respects
new, tendency to use the language and perspective of criminal justice to
articulate demands and to formalise conflicts.

In this chapter I will attempt to analyse the demands for criminalisation
advanced by the so-called 'new' collective actors. This phenomenon,
which takes a specific form in the Italian political context, will, however,
also serve to introduce a more general analysis of a phenomenon, also new
in Italy: namely, the increasing spread of a political and social activism
expressing itself through a language of 'victimisation' (rather than that of
'oppression'). The adoption of the status of victim betrays an indebtedness
to the language and logic of criminal justice, though the relationship with
the criminal justice system itself is by no means central for all such groups
of victims. This shift from the paradigm of oppression to that of 'victimisation' reveals a reconceptualisation of the question of responsibility.

In this chapter I will firstly offer some hypotheses aimed at
understanding why and how collective actors who are bearers of complex
demands refer to the language and logic of the criminal law, and then focus
on what I have called the displacement from oppression to victimisation,
and the various possibilities in the political use of victim status.

SYMBOLIC CRUSADES AND PROCESSES OF CRIMINALISATION

I will begin with three questions: what are the conditions favouring the
emergence of demands for criminalisation; how are these demands to be

understood; and what consequences do they have for the issues which become criminalised and for the forms of self-representation and organisation of the collective actors demanding them?

My object of study here are the demands for criminalisation advanced by collective actors involved in conflicts at least in part aimed at the extension of social and civil rights to groups or areas of life from which they were hitherto excluded. More specifically, I refer to those mobilisations sometimes called 'new social movements': among them, the women's movement and that diverse and fragmented ensemble which goes under the name of environmentalism. To these I will add the mobilisation, of more recent development in Italy, against child abuse. Although this mobilisation appears closer to a traditional 'symbolic crusade' than to a social movement, at least as far as the promoters, the mode of activity and the forms of organisation are concerned, it shares some important characteristics with the first two: it is concerned with civil and social rights; its demands are situated within the same general discourse as feminism and environmentalism[2] and its public is to a large extent the same.

As we have already seen in the previous chapter, the questions which I intend to discuss here lie outside the theoretical programmes and methodologies of contemporary criminology. As far as critical criminology is specifically concerned, though its tradition of research is heavily indebted to the studies of the 'construction of social problems', it too is inadequate to make sense of demands for criminalisation advanced by the very actors with whom the critical criminologist him/herself identifies. This is indicative, of course, of a theoretical weakness. For critical criminology, demands for criminalisation are comprehensible if they can be derived from the interests of dominant social groups, or seen as the result of a translation of 'real' needs into false goals directly or indirectly orchestrated by such groups or, which amounts to the same thing, by the 'logic of the system'. In fact, critical criminology tends to oscillate between positivism and constructionism: a positivistic understanding of the 'dominated' and a constructionist understanding of the 'dominating'. Social problems are social constructions when they are formulated by actors with whom the sociologist does not identify. Such actors are seen – more or less consciously – as driven by interests themselves real in a positivist sense, which the sociologist must reveal. What is false is the problem and what is true are the interests – in domination, maintenance of power – of those who construct the problem. Such interests are usually in conflict with the real needs of the subjects with which the sociologist has chosen to identify her/himself. Even in its more recent versions, such as the new left realism, this criminology has difficulty in making sense of the actor's 'good reasons'. Motivations are deduced: either from class interests or from specific cultural and social circumstances. The actors themselves are reduced to mere impersonations of socio-economic determinations, or atomised into abstract and isolated individuals, as with the category of 'victim'.

The studies of 'symbolic crusades'[3] are among the few which have devoted any attention to the ways in which social demands are constructed, to the relations between types of demands and forms of organisation, between types of demands and the socio-cultural characteristics of the actors mobilising around them, even if in such studies the latter relation is often read in the linear terms of cause and effect. My own thinking differs from that proposed in the existing literature on traditional symbolic crusades in two respects. Firstly the object of study: traditionalist movements and crusades against alcohol, for example, or for the criminalisation of psychotropic drugs, or the campaigns for social purity during the last century, were defensive and oriented to the past, taking the form of the defence of traditional values perceived as threatened by the advance of the new. The mobilisations to which I am referring are, by contrast, oriented to the future: they are 'offensive' (Touraine 1985), in the sense that they struggle for the affirmation of values perceived as new. This distinction has to do with the self-consciousness of the actors involved rather than with the contents, the practice and the consequences of their struggles. However, self-consciousness is a fundamental element, denoting two generally different options, two opposed ways of conceiving oneself and the world.

Secondly, I differ as to the method of approach: the students of symbolic crusades were not directly interested in criminalisation. Rather, while criminalisation was understood as an aim and measure of the success of the majority of these crusades, it was not usually regarded as an issue that merited an analysis in itself. However, questions can be constructed in different ways, and how they are constructed is, as will be seen, significant not only for how the questions themselves come to be perceived but also as an indicator of the internal characteristics of the mobilisation under study. This point alludes to a more fundamental difference from studies of traditional 'moral crusades', that of theoretical and methodological assumptions. In such studies the way in which a question is problematised – whether it is constructed as a medical, political, criminal problem – is either considered irrelevant or treated, generally speaking, as a self evident consequence of the professional interests or socio-cultural characteristics of the actors promoting it. In other words, as if it was the particular way in which the problem is constructed to produce a certain solution.

I propose, instead, to start from the opposite assumption: from the idea that it is the solution which dictates the terms in which the problem is constructed.[4] It is therefore the solution that is the most convenient starting point for inquiry. Such a research strategy is indeed suggested by the movements here under consideration in which the goal of criminalisation does not connect immediately to the professional interests or socio-cultural characteristics of the actors who mobilise around it. The solution 'criminal justice' is not advocated by criminal justice professionals neither is it in any way directly inferable from the culture of the actors demanding it. On the contrary it can be seen as very much in conflict with this same culture, which is rooted in the libertarian and anti-institutional climate of the 1960s and the beginning of the 1970s.

While in the case of most traditional symbolic crusades the resort to criminal law can be seen in the last analysis as a coherent strategy for the defence of those established values for which the crusades were fighting, in the case of the actors with whom I am concerned here such strategy cannot but be more controversial. It takes place, in fact, after twenty years of struggles which have contributed to the delegitimation of the criminal justice system, and which form part of the cultural horizon within which the protagonists of my campaigns move. This situation underlines the need to begin with an interrogation of the solution, criminalisation, and its meanings rather than trying to infer the latter from the aims or cultural milieu of the mobilising movements.

As for the literature on the 'new social movements', it is by now too vast for me to examine here, or even just list. I will refer to that segment of it, by no means internally homogeneous, which sees the question of identity[5] as in some way central to the emergence of contemporary movements (see e.g. Melucci 1985, 1987; Touraine 1988).

But what does 'criminalisation' mean and what does it imply? It does not mean simply the addition of some new forms of behaviour to the already existing list of crimes. It also means that certain activities and situations undergo conceptual and cognitive revision, which in turn implies the creation of a new knowledge around those activities and situations (see Cohen 1988b). The crime of sexual violence already exists in our criminal law. But to conceive as 'sexual violence' a situation in which the characteristic of violence is attributed to, let us say, an abuse of power of a psychological nature means both adding another act to the list of crimes and seeing this action itself in a different way, precisely as a form of sexual violence. To demand the criminalisation of an act implies then to problematise it in a particular way: if the solution to a problem is part of the problem, the criminalising response forms part of the characterisation of that problem to which it is applied. And because the criminalising response is in its very nature a rigid response, allowing no gradations, continuities of evaluation, flexible and elaborate understandings, it transfers these characteristics to the problem, constraining it within these terms. It is therefore of great interest to ask how and why the struggles of collective actors organised around complex issues, such as the liberation of women or the saving and rescue of the natural resources of the planet lead at times – to be sure, in interaction with other groups of actors and their claims – to demands for criminalisation. If, from the standpoint of law and the criminal justice system, such demands signal an accentuation of the use of criminal law as an instrument of social policy, they also have to be studied from the standpoint of the actors which express them.

THE AMBIVALENCE OF CONTEMPORARY MOBILISATIONS

Hitherto I have identified two characteristics which seem to me to be common to the mobilisations I have referred to. One is their orientation to the future, their offensive rather than defensive nature. The other is their character as conflicts oriented to the extension of civil and social rights, characteristics which they share with many other movements of the past. I will argue that the problematisation of the taken for granted is a process inextricably connected to the process of the production of themselves as actors.

What is perhaps new is the content of this self-production, the terrain of conflict, and the forms of organisation. The extension of the area of civil and social rights, in fact, may be a consequence or perhaps one of the objectives of these mobilisations, but that does not exhaust the sense of them. In different ways, the focus of conflict is not simply the inclusion in a system of rights already given, but rather the inclusion in political discourse of questions which challenge this discourse itself. Sexual difference cannot be represented (see e.g. Boccia 1988; Cavarero 1988), it is outside the horizon of the 'social contract'. The 'natural environment' (non-human animals included) presents a similar challenge. The problem of children, at least in Italy, has come to be posed in a way which raises analogous questions. However much, as I will argue in another chapter, the questions posed by the women's movement are irreducible to the problems of other actors mobilised around specific demands, the three cases which I am concerned with here nevertheless have this in common: on one hand they pose typical problems of complex equality (Walzer 1983), on the other they imply a challenge to the ways in which Western culture has understood and theorised its relation to 'nature'. What is ultimately demanded is the recognition as actors of groups excluded from citizenship within the terms of our political and philosophical tradition. (On questions of citizenship in relation to women, see Saraceno 1987; I will return to the issue in the final chapter.)

Many contemporary conflicts, implicitly or explicitly, concern the production of the self, the autonomy of definition and the control of 'identity', the relation with 'nature' (including internal nature).[6] Their terrain is socio-cultural rather than socio-economic. The organisations to which they give rise are in reality often very minimally organised: polycentric, relating to a submerged network of different groups. However, and this is a crucial point, that does not mean that political institutions are not involved in these conflicts, nor that they do not also concern negotiable objectives. It is rather that the ways in which political institutions are confronted, and the struggles for negotiable objectives are directed, are influenced by the non-negotiable horizon within which they are contained. Often, as we shall see, the general orientation and the specific one come into conflict with each other.

THE PRODUCTION OF ONESELF AS ACTOR AND THE CONSTRUCTION OF SOCIAL PROBLEMS

The struggle for the recognition of new rights or for the extension of existing rights to previously excluded groups or situations implies a questioning of normative boundaries and traditional values. It implies, that is, a redefinition of that which hitherto has been considered normal and natural as 'unjust', 'oppressive', 'abnormal' and 'unnatural'. The imputation of injustice or oppression can thus be understood as a move in this struggle, the outcome of which is the production of new knowledge, identification of new fields of research and the construction of new objects of knowledge.

The reconstruction of the 'normal' as a form of 'abuse' implies the attribution of non-natural causes to events and situations. If ecological catastrophies are considered as natural events (and hence inevitable) their causes do not imply any assumption or attribution of responsibility. If we take action because we recognise that birds have a right to live, their death by human hands becomes a condemnable death in which two forms of responsibility are implied. The assumption of responsibility on the part of the defenders of the rights of birds, and simultaneously the attribution of responsibility which these latter impute to those whose actions are considered an assault on these rights. The destruction of the environment which sustains the life of those species of birds is no longer obvious, natural, normal, it is no longer part of the 'order of things': it is an injustice. But as such it gives rise to responsibilities. The problematisation of the obvious, in a word, carries a moral valuation, the attribution of blame. This attribution is at the same time *an imputation and an assumption of responsibility*: actors are constructed at both poles of the process.

The feminist mobilisations of the last twenty years illustrate this process very well. They have produced a new knowledge both in terms of object of cognition and of the mode of cognition itself. This knowledge has denaturalised wide areas of our existence, reconstructing them and presenting them to the general consciousness in a new guise. This is a creative process, in the double sense of creating a new identity and, at the same time, posing new problems and questions. That women occupy a subordinate position with respect to men is a 'fact' documentable across many dimensions. That this fact is however seen as non-natural, unjust, is on the other hand both a driving force for, and a result of the formation of a new collective identity on the part of women. In its turn this imputation of non-naturalness pushes towards the exploration of ever new areas hitherto consigned to the fog of taken-for-grantedness. To repeat, the imputation of injustice, violence, oppression is a move in conflict: it produces both a new consciousness on the part of those who impute and a new understanding of what yesterday was seen as normal and today is defined as oppressive. Denaturalisation and conflict imply the emergence on a previously inanimate scene of actors who are conscious and therefore both responsible and capable of being made to accept that responsibility.

At the same time, this process extends the area of protection and the area of rights. This can be seen in relation to children, the most recent symbolic crusade to reach Italy. To struggle for the extension to children of rights hitherto restricted to adults necessarily involves the critique of adult–child relations hitherto considered normal, or taken for granted. These relations are redefined as liable to violence and abuse of power. A new field of observation is opened and viewed from a new perspective, that of 'the standpoint of children', which renders problematic that which previously was not. In the process of becoming subjects, different groups challenge existing normality, they reconstruct it as historical and therefore change-able, and in introducing conflicts where previously there was peace, they identify new adversaries.[7]

These processes are naturally well known. What however has not been analysed is, as I have said, the relationship between the construction of a problem and its criminalisation. Problems can be constructed in many different ways: as medical, economic, social, cultural etc. The way in which a problem comes to be constructed is inextricably connected with the type of solution which is aimed at and/or which appears available. The attribution of 'causes' is in fact undertaken in the context of the choice of 'solutions'. The latter, in its turn, can be seen as the result of the inter-secting of several factors: the prevalent cultural climate, the relative strength of the actors in conflict, the type of resources at their disposal, their form of organisation, the institutional responses with which they have to contend, their 'world view'.

The key question is therefore that of how we are to understand the present tendency, in the mobilisations I have referred to, to construct problems in criminal terms.[8] What renders the criminal justice solution more attractive and/or more available, than other solutions? An attempt at an answer requires an analysis of both the internal and external context of these mobilisations. An analysis of internal context is necessary because I assume a relationship between the way in which actors construct a problem and both their 'world view' and the organisational imperatives and restrictions within which they operate, since such processes of construction are always the result of conflicts and negotiations. An analysis of the external context is necessary because collective actors operate in a given social, political and cultural environment. Naturally, the internal and external conditions interact with one another.

But even prior to these analyses it is necessary to explore the criminal justice solution itself, what type of solution it is, what it implies, what consequences it can have for the subsequent perceptions and ordering of the problem, and on the self construction of the actors who call for it.

THE CRIMINAL JUSTICE SOLUTION AND ITS CONSEQUENCES

To construct a problem in terms of crime implies the belief that the legal response is the most adequate. But adequate to what objectives? There are three possible ones, mutually interconnected: 1) the diminution of the extent of the problem itself, by means of the threat of punishment and/or the elimination (incarceration) of those responsible. 2) the symbolic acknowledgement of the problem as a universally recognised 'wrong'; and the consequent authoritative legitimation of the imperatives and interests of the instigating group as universal imperatives and interests; 3) the changing of attitudes and dominant cultural norms relating to the problem. These three 'objectives' make reference to three of the functions most commonly attributed to criminal justice: that of general and special prevention; that of the symbolic ordering of protected values in a certain collectivity; that of a pedagogic instrument. Actors can have in mind one or the other of these 'objectives' when they call for the criminalisation of a problem. Whichever they have in mind, however, criminalisation implies all three.

The first objective implies a simplification on both the cognitive and political levels (Cohen 1988b). In order for a problem to be criminalised, it must be defined precisely and rigidly. 'Sexual violence' is 'this' and none other: it is that which the law says it is. Criminalisation selects a situation from within an arc of contiguous situations and events; constructs it as a relationship between two categories of subjects, victim and offender; defines the criteria for the identification of victims and for the identification of offenders, constructs rigidly, that is, the one and the other. To construct the situation as a relationship between victims and offenders, besides implying a cognitive simplification of the problem also implies its political 'reduction' – from a matter of social, economic, medical policy, to one of criminal justice. It means that, if we want to protect victims, we have in the first instance to intervene against offenders. The one and the other lose any other determination and characterisation. From the legal standpoint, ideally, there are neither men nor women, neither rich nor poor, neither black nor white.[9] Criminalisation simplifies, but it also exaggerates and dramatises the conflict. You are either on the side of the offender or on the side of the victim.[10]

In a movement of this type it is not surprising, then, that the struggle for the recognition of some exigencies can adopt the language of the rejection of others. I remember, for example, a conference at Bibbiena in 1982 at which, in the name of female rape victims, the willingness of some (communist) lawyers to act for the defence in rape cases was criticised. Referring to recent campaigns against child abuse, newspaper headlines demanded exemplary punishment for 'monstrous' mothers. And my seven year old niece, brought up to respect plants, 'nature' and above all, animals, could calmly comment, watching the Palio at Siena on television 'if someone has to get hurt, rather the riders than the horses . . .'.[11]

But there is another important aspect to the criminal justice solution which must be recognised. Criminalisation reinforces the individualisation of the attribution of responsibility. Criminal responsibility is personal: to criminalise a problem means imputing it to clearly identifiable individuals, with the consequence that it is only these who will come to be rendered accountable for the problem. The social, political and cultural context, within which the problem occurs and is perceived, tends to disappear into the background. Ecological catastrophies may be, in the last instance, the result of a certain type of economic development; sexual violence the extreme manifestation of domination by one sex over another; child abuse the result of complex social and psychological situations: the process of criminalisation universalises the problem and privatises its 'causes' (but also denaturalises it and we shall see the implications of this later). Criminalisation, while legitimating the problem as a universal concern, individualises the responsibility for it.

As far as the promoters are concerned, criminalisation tends to legitimate their collective 'identity'.[12] When the problem is recognised as crime, their demands are legitimated as universally valid, and they themselves implicitly accepted as political interlocutors. But collective 'identity' established through a process of criminalisation has a double, ambivalent, face. Self-determination and political autonomy are recognised at the same time and as part of the same movement in which the demands for protection are recognised and guaranteed by the state. In this sense the actors present themselves and become accepted as weak subjects, whom the state is obliged to protect by widening the sphere of its intervention in their defence. Self-determination and protection are demands which are often advanced together: they articulate real needs of the demanding groups, but, when these needs are delegated to an extension of legal protection, it becomes more difficult to pass from one to the other. When the demand has been translated into legal terms, the active role of the promoting actors remains inscribed only in the recognition of their demands as worthy of legal protection. Specific actors disappear within the much wider category of victims.

From a political point of view, this leaves room for the legitimation of demands which articulate the need for protection rather than that of self-determination. A recent case, which I will elaborate in greater depth in the last chapter, is that of the events in the Italian parliament during the passage of the bill against sexual violence. Fought for by a section of the women's movement for principled and symbolic motives, the demands for mandatory prosecution, recognition of the gravity of the act of rape, its recognition as violence and not as sex, recognition of women as 'persons' etc., were accompanied by demands for protection – explicit prohibition of interrogation of the victim on aspects of her life not related to the matter under discussion, summary trial. Both in the parliamentary debate and outside parliament the campaign for the Bill found allies on the issue of protection (the presumption of violence in the case of sexual relations between minors or 'handicapped'; the attempt to link the debate on rape to that on pornography etc.) to the detriment of the self-determination aspect. Thus, while the women's movement made use of the discourse of criminal law for its supposed symbolic and pedagogical functions,[13] other groups were able to displace the discussion onto the necessity for greater repression and for a heavier institutional intervention in the private sphere.[14]

This result is further facilitated by the way in which the process of criminalisation fragments a complex problem into linear relations of cause and effect. The abstraction and isolation of a particular aspect of a complex dynamic allows the production of this same aspect as the result of 'causes', other than those proposed by the original actors. In the United States, this process has allowed the convergence in practice between feminist campaigns against sexual violence and pornography and campaigns by the Moral Majority in defence of the 'sanctity of the family'.[15]

THE DEMAND FOR CRIMINALISATION

A complex 'world view', and a political strategy of a potentially similar complexity thus become simplified through the demand for criminalisation. The process of simplification set in motion by the translation of the actors' demands into legal questions is reinforced by successive debates making use of a criminological vocabulary.

In order to develop a hypothesis as to the conditions which make this process possible and attractive, I will analyse first of all the organisational imperatives to which these mobilisations must respond, on the assumption that organisational imperatives, 'world views', and choices of specific objectives are strictly interconnected questions. According to a model elaborated by Douglas and Wildavsky (1983), voluntary groups (in their case ecologically oriented) tend to deal with their organisational imperatives by developing a 'culture of boundaries'. Such a culture is characterised by an orientation to the future; the dramatisation of the present; the construction of 'enemies'; by moral indignation; and by a fundamentalist emotional inspiration.

This model, while it makes the connection between organisational imperatives, world views, and choices of objectives, says nothing as to the conditions of emergence of particular voluntary associations. I refer back therefore to that body of studies on new social movements which focus on the question of 'identity' and which I cited at the beginning. Here the emergence of that particular type of voluntary association to which the mobilisations under examination belong is situated within a more general positioning of conflicts in contemporary Western societies. In these societies, the possibility for actors to participate in the production of their own identities have grown enormously, concomitant, however, with the increase in the potentialities for control and manipulation of this same identity by complex systems. The struggle of actors to appropriate control over the production of their own identity tends to express itself through an appeal to 'nature'. Here, according to this type of study (in particular, Melucci 1987), is located the ambivalence of the new social movements: the reappropriation of identity becomes culturally constructed as a discovery of the non-social. The social is constructed as repressive and manipulative of true internal nature. While such a formulation can contribute to an antagonism towards the apparatuses of regulation and control, it can also lead to the mere celebration of an 'original' identity purified and abstracted from social bonds. The risk is that social movements become closed 'sects'. According to this analysis, the organisational choices depend on the way in which the ambivalence inherent in this 'world view' works itself out in the process of conflict.[16] The impact of these ulterior choices on the 'world view', however, and on the redefinition and choice of specific objectives remains unanalysed.

According to my discussion so far, criminalisation has the following characteristics: it simplifies the objective, radicalises and rigidifies the conflict, it requires and produces a 'friend–enemy' logic. Additionally, it both requires and produces a climate of moral indignation. These characteristics seem coherent with a 'culture of the boundaries' and indicative of a response to the organisational imperatives placed on voluntary organisations. Utilising both the models cited here, we could expect that this will happen when for some reason the ambivalence of contemporary movements gives way to the self-closure into a sect-like organisation.

But criminalisation has other aspects. The simplification of the problem renders it politically negotiable. Additionally, the demand for criminalisation implies the acceptance of the terrain and the rules of conflict as given, it recognises and legitimates the authority of the criminal justice system, it uses official political and legal channels, it delegates the definition and legitimation of its own collective identity to the traditional political institutions. In short, it 'secularises' the relations between movements and institutions, in the context of a reciprocal recognition.

These aspects would seem to cohere rather with what Douglas and Wildavsky (1983) call 'culture of the centre', an expression, in their opinion, of 'hierarchical' or 'market' organisations, oriented towards the past or towards the present. My hypothesis, then, is that demands for criminalisation emerge as the response to organisational imperatives which produce an oscillation between 'culture of the boundaries' and 'culture of the centre'. The demands for criminalisation crystallise these oscillations. If we accept the second model, or the hypothesis that new social movements are structurally ambivalent, we shall be able to understand the demands for criminalisation as attempts to cope with the difficulties of translating this ambivalence into political action in specific circumstances.

Let us take a look now at the context in which the mobilisations have to operate. Such a context is characterised as being constituted by the interaction of multiple actors. First of all, there is the more or less submerged network of groups and individuals to which the networks make reference and by whom they are nourished. Then, the context defined by the traditional political actors, parties, trade unions etc. Then, the institutions and agencies of the state. Another important element is concerned with the quantity and type of resources – economic, cultural, political – which are available. I will not attempt at this point to construct a model which takes account of all these variables. The observation of the changes intervening in the women's movement in Italy during the last fifteen years suggests that when the circumstances lead to a constriction of political space, flexibility and diversification can be perceived as dangerous symptoms of fragmentation and dispersal. The demands for criminalisation can be read then as a type of call to arms: leading to the reconstruction of a collective actor through the identification of a visible enemy. A logic and a rhetoric of the form us/them, accompanied by dramatisation, silences (provisionally) the differences of practice and self consciousness. On one hand the demand for criminalisation dramatises the objective and charges it with emotions deriving their intensity from what the objective itself implicitly refers to, rendering it thereby symbolic of a much more complex situation to which the mobilisations are related. On the other hand, and contemporaneously, criminalisation offers a concrete terrain of struggle, posing itself as an attainable objective.

To summarise my argument: the 'new' mobilisations express complex demands, which imply a relationship between 'culture of the centre' and 'culture of the boundaries' or rather, the consciousness of the necessity to oscillate between the two. These demands are expressions of a diversified, flexible, articulated organisational context, neither hierarchical or sectarian, at least as long as diversification and flexibility are perceived as productive. If there is a restriction of political space and/or the conditions for action change, or the resources utilised for carrying out an ambivalent political practice become reduced, not only can the diversification grow, but it can also be perceived as dangerous for the maintenance of the collective identity constructed up to that point. Demands for criminal-isation can then emerge as re-unifying motives on the organisational level and at the same time as the symbols of a non-forgotten ambivalence.

Naturally, when the political space is reduced by the recourse to a politics and rhetoric of 'emergency' and 'public order', the use of the symbolic potential of criminal justice becomes even more attractive. And this is what happened, not only in Italy, during the last twenty years. The crisis of the culture of the welfare state – the terrain of growth of radical and complex demands – has had many consequences on this level: dis-appointment and distrust in the institutional responses; a contradictory impulse to re-privatise social problems which has led to the formulation of fragmented and sectoralised demands, often formulated in terms pre-constituted by the practice and logic of institutional agencies;[17] a consensual politics based on campaigns of moral panic, with the double effect of restricting the access of non-traditional actors to the political scene and reducing the language of politics to one of 'war'.

In a climate already marked culturally by the dominance of a political discourse of public order, a campaign can produce criminalising effects even when these are not explicitly contemplated by the actors of the campaign itself. This is the case with the present campaign against child abuse. But this occurs also because many of the elements which 'favour' criminalisation are already present within the campaign: the isolation of the problem, and its simplification into a problem of the relationship between brutal adults and defenceless children; a certain indifference to the context in which such brutality is produced; the emphasis on victimisation. As emblematic of the changes in the cultural climate from the 1970s to the present I would cite only one example: the episode, reported in the Italian newspapers, of the prostitute mother who tied her nine year old son to the bed when she had to go out to work at night. A situation which, at least in the liberal press, would have been described some years ago as a problem of poverty, neglect, lack (perhaps culpable lack) of adequate social work intervention, besides being a symptom of a generally 'unjust' society, today is portrayed by this same medium, as an episode of savage brutality, in which there is only one person clearly responsible and guilty: the mother. Such an account both presupposes and reinforces some of the characteristics of the criminalising response.

FROM OPPRESSION TO VICTIMISATION

The question of identity is central to what here has been defined as ambivalence. Hitherto I have used the term 'collective identity' in an intuitive way. If we try to analyse it a little more closely, we see that collective identity has at least two aspects. The first refers to the recognition of the group as collective actor, as political subject; the other has to do with the project and the construction of a common identity. The two aspects are obviously interconnected, but can also enter into conflict. The struggle to be recognised as political actors can conflict with the internal process of constructing a common identity: again, the example of the women's movement is the clearest. The project of an identity based on the elaboration of sexual difference contrasts with demands which carry a notion of sexual difference as a result of the processes of victimisation, and which therefore adopt the very philosophical and political language of 'equality' (and of rights) which the project of sexual difference seeks to subvert (Vega 1988). I will postpone a further exploration of these themes until the last chapter.

If the relationship between the two types of collective identity is particularly problematic for certain actors[18] and less for others, to entrust the recognition of one's own political identity to the criminal justice system carries for all the difficult relationship between self-determination and protection. This difficult relationship is consigned to the designation of self as victim. The status of autonomous political actor becomes derived from the 'recognition' of one's common situation as victims.

I would like to confront here an aspect relating to the increased recourse to the utilisation of the symbolic potential of criminal justice already noted in the previous chapter: there is nowadays a growing protagonism of 'victims'; rather, we may note an increased use of this self-designation of 'victim' to legitimate one's political presence and activity. It is notably the self-definition as 'victim of crime' which has seen a new fortune: a fact which signifies, in my opinion, a significant distancing from the semantic field implied by the notion of 'oppression'. Oppression referred to a composite condition, relatively stable over time, the result of different factors, only some of which could be theorised as intentional actions. Victimisation, by contrast, refers to a simple situation which is the outcome of precise, intentional actions and which includes only those actors who are the objects of 'victimising' actions. The category of oppression is omnicomprehensive, denoting every aspect of identity and every sphere and mode of action, it understands the past as collective history and identifies actors 'heavy' with constraints. The category of victimisation instead translates collective history into individual biography (though sometimes symbolic of a collective biography), and emphasises a single aspect of this biography; the actors which it constructs are the abstract subjects of law, the subjects entitled to the fundamental rights relating to life, liberty and property. From this point of view, we might say that the language of victimisation articulates traditional liberal concerns, whereby the language of oppression legitimated not only socialist but social-democratic concerns at the basis of the welfare state.

Victimisation has become a crucial question both for the so-called conservative criminologies and sociologies as well as the critical tradition; the object of a relatively new discipline, victimology; the legitimation and/or the inspiration for new social and criminal justice policies and, in Italy at least, the terrain for the constitution of groups and associations active on the political scene. I would like to utilise the self-attribution of victim status by the social movements that I have described, to advance some hypotheses about the meaning of the present centrality of a discourse on victimisation.

The displacement of attention from 'criminals' to their victims both within the sociological literature and in public debate has already been noted (Lasch 1984; Cohen 1988b). It has been read as a reaction, both in radical and conservative circles, to the excessive attention to the misfortunes of the 'criminals' prevalent during the 1960s. I have already noted how within critical criminology for example, both the abolitionists and the new left realists, from apparently opposite sides, converge on the proposal to reintroduce the victim into the complex relationship defined as crime. I would argue rather that what we are witnessing is not so much a shift of focus – from the centrality (of the problems) of 'criminals' to that of their victims – but a complex semantic mutation which has political and theoretical implications of vast import. As I have already argued in the previous chapter, it was the criminals who were seen as victims, at least in the 'left' sociological literature of the 1960s and the early years of the 1970s. Of what they were victims and how far such victimisation was held 'responsible' for the commission of crimes depended to a large extent on the ideological starting point of the sociologist. Within radical sociology, I noted, offenders were held to be victims both of the logic and selective practices of the criminal justice system and of the unjust, oppressive circumstances in which they lived. Here, victimisation was seen, rather than as the result of action, as a process and a condition relating to the subjective experience of socio-structural factors. The terminology of oppression described both the subjective experience and its social roots. Whether it was self-assumed, or, more often, attributed, the label of victim characterised the individual result of a collective situation. Criminals were victims if and when theirs was not a collectively undertaken action ('organised' crime, 'white collar' crime, and crimes of the 'powerful' were usually examined through different categories); a status of relative autonomy was allocated to criminals (rather like the state . . .); while in general an instrumental rationality was admitted in their actions, responsibility was broadly distributed: to social circumstances, to the criminal justice system, to the lack of legitimate opportunities, to broken families, etc.

The characteristics of this literature have already been analysed. What I wish to argue is that we are witnessing not a simple shift in emphasis, from the misfortune of the criminals to that of their victims – something which might after all be characterised as an act of redistributive justice. Rather, we are witnessing a shift from the semantic field associated with oppression to the semantic field associated with victimisation. In the sociological literature on criminality and its control this shift runs in parallel with a more general shift in the perception of victims. In tracing the history of the discovery of child abuse, for example, Pfohl (1977) notes that while initially this discovery led to a taking of responsibility for the children themselves (through institutionalisation, entrustment to foster families, etc.), today it leads to an intervention oriented towards those responsible for the abuse (in the form of treatment, criminalisation, etc.). If the emphasis on offenders as victims implied putting 'society' on trial as oppressive and the imperative to 'look after' the criminals; the emphasis on the victims of crime implies the putting on trial of criminality as such and the imperative to control criminals, or potential criminals, in an efficient way.[19] As has been seen in the previous chapter, the present direction of critical criminology does not seem to be conscious of this change. It tends to work in terms of a simple inversion: up to a few years ago we thought that it was the criminals who were oppressed, now we see that also (certain types of) victims are oppressed, besides being victimised. The latter being doubly oppressed, it is their standpoint that has to be adopted. This project is not, however, adhered to: adopting the standpoint of the victims can only mean recognising them as actors when they define themselves as such (whatever doubts one might have about whether they are also 'oppressed') and being disposed to understand the category of victim as socially constructed. In general, however, victims are identified on the simple basis of having suffered a crime, treated as distinct individuals and abstracted from the social and cultural context from which they borrow the necessary vocabulary to describe themselves as victims.

What is most striking today is precisely the presence on the contemporary political scene of collective actors who define themselves as victims. There are by now many groups and associations constructed on the basis of a common recognition of themselves as victims of crime: it is sufficient to cite the victims of the mafia and terrorism. It is a temporary basis, which cuts across class, gender, age and occupation. Other groups, including the mobilisations I have been concerned with here: the women's movement, the environmentalists, the campaigners against child abuse, have chosen, at a certain moment, to present themselves as victims of crime, or have selected and reconstructed a particular aspect of their own condition, or the condition of those on whose behalf they act, in such a way as to adapt it to this definition.

There are then at least three aspects worthy of note in the shifting of interest from offenders to victims; the semantic change in the notion of victim; the emergence of 'victims' as collective actors on the political scene (that is, an increase in the use of this label by collective actors as a way of legitimating their own demands); the centrality of the criminal justice system and of a criminological vocabulary in the definition of victim.[20]

According to Lasch (1984), this diffusion of the self-assumption of victim status corresponds to an increasing perception of impotence, derivable, in its turn, from certain characteristics of 'consumer society'. Certainly, if we relate the decline in the 'discourse of oppression' to the conditions of emergence of this feeling of impotence we grasp, perhaps, one aspect of the question. The discourse of oppression implies the possibility of radical social change, the authors of which are precisely the oppressed themselves. However, as we have seen, this discourse has another aspect. To the interpretation I called omnipotent there corresponds an impotent one, with paradoxical results: the extension of the sphere of the social has involved the dispersal of the imputation of responsibility. Where society in its totality is held responsible for 'injustices', no particular individual or group of individuals is called to account. The dominant sociological literature, whether of Marxist or systemic orientation, has at the same time told this story and reinforced such an interpretation. In such a context the self-attribution of victim status cannot be seen only as the translation of diffused feelings of impotence into a category descriptive of 'reality'. I would instead argue that the adoption of a criminological vocabulary is, at least in part, indicative of a reaction to a paradoxical de-subjectivisation. The new centrality of the criminal justice system, the abnormal increase in recourse to it as a way of legitimating interests, marking out conflicts, confirming values – a recourse which is thus charac-terised by the utilisation of the symbolic potential of criminal justice – must be (also) understood as an attempt to use it as a site in which action is redefined as intentional, where the process of indictment refers precise facts and events to clearly identified actors to whom are attributed 'con-sciousness and free will'. The collective adoption of victim status thus has to be seen in the context defined by increasing recourse to the symbolic potential of criminal justice, a recourse which speaks of an attempt to reintroduce actors onto the social stage.

That these actors, be they offenders or victims, do not seem to possess other characteristics besides those of 'consciousness' and 'will', or that what distinguishes them is the fact that they act intentionally, is an ulterior indicator of this attitude. It seems possible to detect, in the processes of criminalisation here under consideration, a sort of ironic consciousness that what one is doing is precisely reimposing 'actors' onto a confused and undifferentiated scenario: in order to recognise consciousness and will in 'us', it is first of all necessary to attribute consciousness and will to 'others'. The social determinants are not so much forgotten as put in parenthesis. The awareness of their existence remains, but it is seen as necessary to leave them out of consideration. The actor who emerges from the demand for criminalisation is not 'weak' as a result of being determined in various ways, but rather abstracted from his/her own determinations, constructed as signifying the existence of a conflict, rather than personally involved in that conflict. However real the consequences, for all the actors involved, of the processes of criminalisation, the latter have a prevalently symbolic nature.[21]

The slippage from a discourse of oppression to one of victimisation can then be seen as indicative of a more general emergence and diffusion of 'voice' (Hirschman 1982): actors having in common only the experience of being victims, engage in a plurality of conflicts aimed at populating the political stage with clearly identified antagonists. This in turn is a precondition for they themselves to become recognised and legitimated as actors. The criminal justice system is the privileged arena in which responsibility is assumed and attributed in public, symbolic forms recognisable by all.

DIFFERENT WAYS OF BEING VICTIMS

In the United States the movement for Victim's Rights has not enjoyed a good press on the left, at least recently. It has in fact been accused, even by those who have been among the first to support, recognise and study victim problems (see Viano 1987), of lending itself to co-option by conservative law and order campaigns which, in the name of the rights of victims, call for types of crime control which are repressive, 'incapacitating' and above all injurious to the rights of the accused.[22] Other, more complex and differentiated aspects of this movement remain however unexplored, even, for example, in the investigation of moral crusades like that organised by MADD (Mothers Against Drunken Driving) (see Reinarman 1988). This movement was certainly responsible for the passage of repressive legislation towards motorists caught driving after having drunk (even relatively modest quantities of) alcohol. But, otherwise, as a movement it was indicative of the organising capabilities, the political ability, the enterprising ability of 'mothers' and, more generally, as I said before, of the tendency to assume responsibility, in addition to and alongside attributing responsibility.

How modes of assumption and attribution of responsibility are interconnected and how they result in different political configurations and actors of differing status, I will seek to illustrate with three Italian cases which exemplify three different modes of understanding oneself as a victim and of orienting oneself to state and criminal justice institutions.

The first example I have already in part illustrated, and I will refer to it again more generally in the last chapter of this book: namely the women's movement and the law on sexual violence. As I have already said, here the assumption of victim status has above all a symbolic significance. It has the meaning of proclaiming and establishing one's innocence (a very political gesture towards a culture that holds women responsible for their own violation) and of constructing themselves as (abstract) bearers of rights. At a double cost: the loss of the sexual and gendered character of rape; the construction of actors (the victims) as acted upon rather than agents, a construction which the criminal justice system tends to confirm (see Vega 1988). Worse, the construction of oneself as a mere bearer of rights implies denying the possibility of being recognised as full subjects *qua women*.

That women are conscious of the double bind constituted by the struggle for a decent law on sexual violence is testified by the debate on prosecution, wanted by some to be mandatory and by others to be victim-initiated. The issue was constructed in terms of 'female liberty'. The supporters of mandatory prosecution, as I have noted, argued that this freedom must be identical to that proclaimed and defended by the entire political community in the case of any serious crime. Conversely, that the equating of rape to any other serious crime signified the full admission of women to the political community. The supporters of victim-initiated proceedings argued that female liberty cannot be reduced to or made homologous with the liberty protected by the criminal law, because the present legal system is a 'mono-gendered' (male) structure and the admission of women to the political community occurs to the extent to which they become considered as men. Victim-initiated proceedings, on the other hand, by implying the necessity to create the conditions in which the individual woman is in a position to freely decide whether or not to report the offence, would place female liberty within the construction of 'a common world of women', rather than entrust it to the homologising abstract institutional protection.

I anticipate here some of the considerations that I will elaborate further on. If criminal justice is utilised for its symbolic potential, the position of mandatory prosecution is stronger, because it is coherent with the abstract and neutral notion of victim. Conversely, it is precisely this neutrality and abstractness which sustains the necessary innocence of the victims. Since it is this innocence that the adoption of victim status establishes, and since this adoption, in the determinate context of criminal justice, constructs the victimising event as something that occurs between two rigidly separate parties, and solely characterised by the innocence (and passivity) of the one and by the culpability (and activity) of the other, there does not seem to me to remain much space for the affirmation of a female liberty, defined by the difference of sex. The problem, here, is not then that of 'female liberty', but of a 'self-determination' conceived in the abstract terms of our liberal political tradition (see again Vega 1988). The demands for criminalisation reintroduce actors, but, I repeat, simple actors; and when one part of them is constructed as victims, their capacity for action remains confined to the same process of criminalisation. Once this has been exhausted, the criminalising collective actors vanish as collective actors and assume the individual and passive role of victims.

The second example concerns the associations of the victims of terrorism (right wing terrorism, probably because such terrorism is more oriented to 'massacres' of innocent bystanders and a single bomb can be responsible for the killing and wounding of many people).[23] These associations were born as a reaction to what was perceived as the delays, the inertia, the disinterest (at times due to complicity) on the part of the state in carrying out investigations and prosecuting those responsible. They are 'single issue' associations, the members of which have nothing else in common other than having been victims or relatives of the victims of terrorist acts. They act outside the traditional political organisations and organise themselves on the basis of informal, face to face, relations (see Turnaturi, Donolo 1988). They choose as their interlocutors primarily the various criminal justice agencies (police, judiciary etc.), but conduct investigations themselves, pressuring the mass media, keeping contacts and stimulating the intervention of the political parties. As parties to civil action for damages arising from criminal cases, they obviously have an important part in the proceedings.

In cases like this, the adoption of victim status has made possible a form of political activity – outside the traditional political organisations – of groups of 'private' citizens; it has given them a very effective voice, the more effective the more it is seen as the articulation of sufferings directly experienced. It is precisely this rendering public of private grief, a rendering public that remains as a matter of policy the property of those who suffer it, which makes these associations such a new phenomenon on the Italian scene (Turnaturi, Donolo 1988). By making the political and judicial institutions directly responsible for their own actions and omissions towards the sufferings endured, the participants in these associations assume responsibility, not as members of a political organisation, nor as bearers of some official mandate, but precisely as 'private' citizens, whose problems both remain private and become public preoccupations.[24] Two types of responsibility are called for by them: on one hand they underline criminal responsibility (for example pursuing the indictment of terrorist suspects and opposing decarceration measures for the convicted), on the other hand, by demanding institutional reparation and compensation for damage, they call for a process of collective responsibilisation towards what they suffered. The two types are connected because the first, which implies the utilisation of and the passage through the criminal law, establishes their having been victimised and thus the fact that they are deserving of compensation (which among other things, if it were not already obvious, shows that contemporary issues of responsibility emerge within a culture of social rights: the imputation of individual responsibility does not cancel, indeed it often reinforces, demands for collective responsibilisation directed to the state and its institutions. (On analogous themes see Abel 1982c; Gusfield 1975.))

The third example is in reality double. It concerns the associations of relatives of the mentally ill, which have arisen during the last fifteen years after the enactment of psychiatric reform law 180 of 1978. This law, about which I shall say more later, has highlighted numerous and interconnected questions of responsibility: the complex responsibility of psychiatric workers; the new responsibility of psychiatric patients, to whom civil rights have been restored; the responsibility of the families and of other support networks in the face of the impossibility of forced hospitalisation and long term confinement (at least in public hospitals). The context within which these associations move is thus constituted by the local psychiatric services, the local authorities, the political organisations and national institutions. The criminal justice system is not involved except peripherally – being utilised to identify or dramatise dysfunctions, to pursue conflicts between different agencies (we shall give an example of this in the next chapter) – but not, primarily, to assume the status of victim. They share with the associations of the victims of terrorism the fact of being spontaneous aggregations, autonomous from the political parties, arisen on the basis of private problems. They may make use of or work with experts, but their authority and influence does not derive from some specific knowledge, but rather from the fact that their members are directly involved in the problems with which they are concerned. In other words, they maintain full control of what they complain about. There are many such associations (see for a summary and description, Giannichedda 1987) differing in respect of organisation, objectives, activity. Some are basically pressure groups, working for a revision to the law generally along the lines of a reintroduction of some type of custodial institution. The majority of such groups work on various levels for the full implementation of the same law through negotiation and conflict with the medical services and local authorities, often working with them for the development of alternative projects, providing information, acting as support networks.

It is possible to identify two different ways of understanding the status of victim in this case because here this status is assumed in the context of a conflict between clients and services. For the associations which behave as pressure groups, victims are above all the psychiatric patients. Here victim indicates a condition of absolute impotence and complete determination: psychiatric patients are ill, therefore they are not only not responsible for their condition, but not even able to take decisions regarding it. It is therefore demanded that they become the complete responsibility of the social and medical services whether they desire it or not. For the other type of association, victim describes both the situation of the patients and that of their relatives: it does not construct a condition of absolute impotence, but rather a condition which is the result of the unjust and incorrect handling of the problem on the part of the social and medical services and more generally the public bodies concerned. The adoption of this status has thus the significance of making visible the desire to be recognised as interlocutors by services and public institutions thereby becoming the principal and directly interested party to the question: which means that while responsibility is attributed it is also assumed, and the non-formal recognition of this assumption is demanded.

There are many ways, then, of assuming and acting out the status of victim. When in this definition the criminal is a central element, it has different consequences if those who claim it for themselves are a collective actor moving within a horizon of complex issues, or if they are a single-issue collective actor whose very existence depends precisely on this definition. In the context of social services and institutions, different consequences occur if the merit worthiness of the victim is made dependent on his/her innocence (and passivity) or on his/her 'right' to be considered an interlocutor.

'VICTIMS' AND THE POLITICS OF RIGHTS

I said that the shift from oppression to victimisation indicates a more diffuse and general access to 'voice'. This access takes the form of a demand for ever new rights. The demand for rights signals the constitution of new actors on the social and political scene. Vice versa, through their appeal for rights these new actors demand to be accorded the status of full legal subjects or, to use a different terminology, to be recognised as fully citizens.

The scenario of criminal justice, I have argued so far, is attractive precisely because it offers a reconstruction of actors. Such actors, I also said, are abstract actors, characterised by nothing else apart from their ability to 'know and will': i.e., from their being *a priori* endowed with a freedom that signifies absolute independence and self-sufficiency. Any constraint to, or qualifications of, this self-sufficiency is constructed as subtracting from this freedom, as constituting an impediment to it. Such reconstruction appears then to happen through recourse to a classical liberal rhetoric used against what I called the paradoxical desubjectivisation operated by the welfare state. Thus, the self-attribution of a victim status is not so much a statement of impotence as, on the contrary, a means to action.

It is action that takes place within the context of welfare institutions and arises and is inspired by a diffuse culture of not only civil and political, but also social, rights. Women, children, relatives of the mentally ill, mothers of drug addicts, victims of crime and terrorism do not, in general, call for a retreat of state intervention: on the contrary, they ask for a qualified intervention, that can be made accountable, and such as to enhance rather than mortify their status as citizens. This demand is in contradiction to recourse to the language of criminal justice, and is not met by the mere recognition of one's status as full legal subject. Many argue that it is in contradiction to the very language and policies of rights (see, for example, Minow 1990; Wolgast 1991), in that the standard subject of rights is the abstract, self-sufficient, self-contained (Hirschman 1992), independent individual (I shall come back on this in the last chapter). Welfare social policies, or policies that try to foster substantive equality have been on the one hand often in contrast with civil liberties, and on the other have reproduced 'differences' (i.e., all that differs from the standard subject of rights) as inequalities.

But at the same time that these actors recur to criminal justice or adopt a victim status to merely signify agency and invoke rights, they stay on the social and political scene as concrete, 'embedded' actors: as women, mothers of drug addicts, relatives. It is true that many of these groups constitute themselves on the basis of each member defining herself as a 'victim': but in so doing each member does not abdicate all other characteristics. On the contrary, we see mothers of drug addicts, relatives of the mentally ill, sisters or wives or fathers of victims of terrorism. In other words, these are individuals ('victim' is an individualising label) who assume responsibility on the basis and in the context of their relationships. They do not claim rights as abstract, self-sufficient subjects, but as (individual) members of families. The same may be said of women, children, ethnic minorities insofar as they demand recognition of an 'embedded' self. The articulation of these demands in terms of 'rights' may have the paradoxical result of a misrecognition of precisely that embeddedness, or of its recognition at the expense of one's status as an individual (as in the case of ethnic minorities). In the next chapters I shall describe a similar problem in the case of minors and the mentally sick in their relationship with criminal justice.

What, however, I want to signal here, is that many of those individuals acting together on the basis of having been individually wronged as members of families may be seen to give a new meaning to citizenship. From the mere entitlement to rights, the fuller the more closely one resembles the standard subject of rights, to the discharge of a responsibility which is assumed both towards oneself and one's family and towards society as a whole.

I am then hypothesising a further shift: from the politics of victimisation to a politics of what I am going to call 'sovereignty' (I shall dwell on this more in the last chapter), that challenges both traditional welfare policies and classical liberal ones, by posing the problem of the full recognition of an embedded subject.

I will argue in the last chapter that (a certain kind of) women's politics may be taken as the paradigm of this politics. The symbolic potential of criminal justice would be of little use in it; on the other hand, the language, logic, and mode of operation of criminal justice may be fruitfully criticised from its point of view.

5 The question of juvenile deviance

Juveniles, mentally ill, women, constitute – in different ways – the principal 'exceptions' (which confirm the rule) for the criminal justice system. They are exceptions with separate histories, especially as regards the institutions and knowledges through which they have been constructed and to whose care they have been delegated (though in all three cases a relevant role is and has been played by the institutions and knowledges of psychology and psychiatry). They nevertheless have in common precisely this: that they make evident how modern law (and rights) arise historically, are constructed by and pertain predominantly to the male, adult citizen, to whom is attributed the full capacity to distinguish good from evil and to orient his behaviour as a consequence. These three characteristics are clearly interconnected. Only to the adult male is attributed the type of rationality which has become the paradigm of rationality in general, being constructed on the experience and interests of (certain) male adults.

The exceptions to such rationality are the privileged terrain of the non-juridical knowledges, the so-called human sciences, both in a supporting relation to law, and in conflict with it, using the exceptions to construct paradigms and institutions which tend to erode the 'rule' itself. In both cases the task of these sciences has been to argue a lack of rationality – or rather to explore the conditions which limit or eliminate a responsibility perceived as the innate property of the individual – and to identify modalities distinct from criminal justice to control, prevent and repress undesirable attitudes and behaviours.[1]

I do not intend, in this chapter, to retrace the history of juvenile justice (for the Italian case see De Leo 1981). I am concerned rather to extract from this history an aspect which seems to me particularly indicative of current attitudes, in Italy, towards the relationship between criminal justice and juridical knowledge on the one hand and other modes of control, cure, care, and psycho-sociological knowledge on the other. This aspect is specifically related to the debate on two of the types of judgements most frequently delivered by (Italian) juvenile court judges in order to release juveniles accused of criminal acts: the 'judicial pardon' and the judgement of 'immaturity'. In this debate the question of the punishability of non-adults is clearly articulated as a field of distinct options within criminal justice and social policy. In this field various bodies of knowledge and institutions interact and conflict and a multiplicity of orientations, preoccupations and interests can be found which make more general reference to the themes of public order in so-called 'post-welfare' societies.

A DIFFERENT JUSTICE

The modern status of non-adult (see Ariès 1974) as that of non-male, is characterised in terms of its non-normality. It is not simply a question of different conditions but rather conditions that diverge from an assumed standard of universal measure: anything which diverges from this standard is already for that very reason close to pathology.

Youth has become, in modern times, a distinct condition, denoted by contradictory attributes: it is an increasingly longed-for condition, a value in itself, while at the same time it is characterised by social marginality and prolonged economic dependence. It is a problem in itself: site of innovation and authenticity but also of uncertainty, precariousness and risk.

Not simply incomplete adults, and yet characterised by a 'difference' understood in terms of 'lack', juveniles are the objects of a system of justice whose difference and separateness from that of adults is justified by reference to an ideology of protection anchored in a body of theories regarding the nature of infancy and adolescence. It is precisely this that has made so-called 'delinquency' a privileged object of psychological and sociological study in the Anglo-Saxon literature, a paradigm for the construction of a sociology of deviance – and an otherwise privileged field for experimentation in judicial and penal policies later often applied to adults.

The modern social status of juveniles, characterised by economic, emotional and legal dependence, is justified in terms of a supposed lack of adult capacities – maturity of judgement, self-control, self-determination. This in turn legitimises a system of justice based around 'needs' rather than 'rights'. This view of juvenile justice produces studies of the psychological and social causes, not only of transgressions of the criminal law but also of attitudes and conducts which would not be stigmatised or considered problematic among adults (leaving home, sexual promiscuity, family conflicts, etc.): or, all those forms of behaviour which can be construed, in the terminology of the Italian penal code, as 'irregularity of conduct and character'.

I will be concerned in this chapter only with the penal aspect of juvenile justice. However, the strictly penal aspect is not only supposedly inspired by a different logic to that of the adult criminal justice system, but is also closely interrelated with administrative and welfare aspects. This inter-relation is currently a terrain of uncertainties and institutional conflicts. Two opposed tendencies converge in pushing towards a separation of functions, towards the division of tasks between penal juvenile justice and welfare agencies: the one concerned with the conversion of individual needs into social rights; the other stressing the necessity of social defence.

The interrelation between welfare and punishment is however the *raison d'être* of juvenile justice, that which legitimises its separate existence. The interrelation between protection and punishment, between intervention with 'educative' aims and segregation with the aim of 'correction', imple-mented in different ways in successive periods, characterises the definition and administration of the juvenile condition – and in particular that of the economically and socially marginalised, juvenile poor – from the stand-point of justice. Up until not long ago some form of institutionalisation seemed the adequate response to any problem: transgression of criminal laws, 'irregularity of conduct and character', family inadequacies, prob-lems of educational achievement, etc.

Authoritative intervention resulting in institutionalisation aimed not at 'correction' or punishment, but at protection, education, and removal from negative family and environmental influences was justified and legitimated in terms of the 'good' of children. Both in the past and in the present such intervention and institutionalisation are more frequent in the case of young females than in that of males, in areas where criminal acts are not involved, such as running away from home, sexual promiscuity, disobedience towards the family, or in the case of family contexts or environments which are considered unhealthy. (For a bibliography see Faccioli, Pitch 1988. An Italian literature as rich as the Anglo-Saxon one still does not exist, see however Buttafuoco 1985; Groppi 1983–4.)[2]

The notion of difference elaborated in terms of lack or deficit of 'rationality' (in the case of juveniles provisional, in the case of women permanent) is precisely what justifies interventions in the name of needs rather than rights. The definition and articulation of needs is entrusted to adults in general, and in particular to the various experts who, over the last century, have competed for and subdivided scientific competence on infancy, adolescence, and most recently 'youth'. The social history of interventions in defence of the so-called weak sections of the population is a complex one, not understandable simply as a story of colonisation, discrimination or the portraying of a particular group as inferior. Neither is it a linear process without conflicts and contradictions.

It has nevertheless almost always had a particularly ambiguous and potentially 'heavy' side in the area of punishment. When protection is justified in terms of inadequacy or need, punishment is justified by the necessity of, and the opportunity for, correction; or, by the existence of dangerousness. In both cases, whether for the good of the juvenile or that of society, it operates through the attenuation or suspension of those legal safeguards accorded to adults. In Italy, due to the influence of the positivist school (De Leo 1981), the juvenile who has committed crimes and is declared not liable may be subjected to security measures[3] such as referral to a reformatory. The deficit of rationality, biological and psychological abnormality – just as in the case of the mentally ill accused of criminal acts – are seen as connected (though today no longer automatically, see next chapter) with social dangerousness.

DELINQUENCY IN ITALY

If juvenile justice, its practices and institutions have been and are, objects of political and social debate, much less interest is aroused by transgressive behaviour on the part of young people as such (see De Leo, Cuomo 1983). Crimes connected to terrorism and drug addiction have raised questions about the social and cultural status of the protagonists, but these last have been usually young people over eighteen years old (therefore, adults, as far as the law is concerned). It would seem that Italy is not, nor has ever been in a relevant way, touched by analogous phenomena to those which have given rise to a flourishing American (predominantly) and English literature: delinquent gangs (Cohen 1955), petty criminality etc., seen as conduct typical of the condition of youth in large urban ghettos, with whom, by means of the term 'delinquency', are associated acts and be-haviours which are 'deviant' but not illegal (running away from home, truancy, having illegitimate children etc.). Whether this is a real difference or the product of a different way of interpreting and constructing the problems, the Italian literature on this theme tends to restrict itself to an examination of the institutional aspects of the question. This is the case for both the sociologists and criminologists,[4] and all the more so for the professionals in juvenile justice, judges, psychologists, social workers, educators. It is indeed these latter who are the principal protagonists of the debate on 'delinquency': in Italy, delinquency is thus constructed as an institutional question rather than as a social problem or rather, as a social problem which immediately evokes and is inextricably related to, the policies and practices of management, care and solution.[5]

It is thus a debate whose difference with respect to the Anglo-Saxon literature testifies both to the difference of the phenomenon and to that of the forms of definition and management, notwithstanding some apparent similarities of language, legitimating ideology and the penetration and use in Italy from the 1960s onwards, of interpretative models imported from the Anglo-Saxon context. The academic literature and the political debate on juvenile delinquency reveal the peculiarities already noted, for Italy, in relation to the issue of crime in general: in particular, the weight of contributions by professionals in the area, who make themselves, with greater or less awareness, subject and object of the analysis. The result is the production of investigations of the juvenile justice system which are critical, but as they are internal to this system itself, they never question precisely its being a different and separate system.

From a different standpoint, the contributions of the professionals can be read as indicative of the interests, orientations and problems relative to their own distinct competences; and indicative of the conflicts among these different competences themselves. The situation which the debate here under discussion takes as its background presents contradictory aspects which are not easy to interpret (see Faccioli 1988, 1988a).

In an article in 1977 Tullio Bandini interpreted the decline in reported, tried and convicted juvenile offences, in the context of a general increase in crime and of a rise in the number of preventive detentions, as the result of a generalised feeling of failure and impotence on the part of professionals – judges in particular – resulting in an unprogrammed depenalisation. Such depenalisation was a partial and contradictory process, punctuated by repressive moments, as the increased use of preventive detention showed. Ten years later (see Faccioli 1988: the data analysed refer to the years 1976–85), reported offences appear to be still falling but convictions are rising while at the same time the use of incarceration is falling. The increase in convictions, significant as it is, does not cancel out the much higher percentage of acquittals in relation to the total juveniles sentenced: more than 80 per cent of juveniles brought before the courts are acquitted, in large measure due to the concession of judicial pardon (almost 60 per cent of acquittals). As far as custodial detentions are concerned, they are falling extensively both in number and in terms of length of sentence, but the percentage of male juveniles detained after conviction has doubled over the last decade (from 3 to 6 per cent) (see also De Stroebel 1985). Juveniles are overwhelmingly reported (73 per cent), convicted (71 per cent) and incarcerated (82 per cent) for crimes against property: largely theft and robbery. There has also been a diminution in the rate of release on parole (Fadiga, Gerratana, Occulto 1985).

Increase in sentences, reduction in the use of detention; high rate of acquittal, reduction in the use of parole. Even taking into account relevant local differences, the operation of juvenile justice appears during the last ten years particularly contradictory. The tendency towards decarceration, noticeable since the 1970s, continues to prevail (reinforced by the net reduction in the use of security measures), and nevertheless the steep climb in the number of convictions and the reluctance to use parole, which cannot be explained in terms of a change in the nature of offences for which juveniles are appearing in court, indicates, as I will seek to argue, the deepening of the crisis of functionality of juvenile justice and the attempts by judges to confront it.

FROM CORRECTION TO RE-EDUCATION

The picture described above is further complicated by the data on juveniles committed to institutions under administrative and civil measures (see below). According to the statistical institute ISTAT, between 1980 and 1985 there was an increase in the number of young people of both sexes in re-educative institutions; according to information by the Ministry of Justice, on the contrary, only in Sicily, a region of special status where law 616 of 1977 (which delegates the implementation of administrative (care and cure) measures to local authorities) is not in force, though there are still juveniles in these institutions their numbers are declining (see Faccioli 1988). Faccioli propounds two hypotheses to explain this contradiction. According to the first, it is simply the fact that ISTAT includes under the category of admission to re-educative institutions juveniles under administrative and civil measures (care and cure), which would mean that these young people were not effectively institutionalised. In the second hypothesis, the data register the effective presence of juveniles in re-educative institutions due to scarcity, particularly in certain localities, of other solutions.

Administrative measures refer to the activity of juvenile courts with regard to young people considered 'irregular in conduct and character' – young people that is, who are not charged with offences, but with transgressions which would not be such if committed by adults: indiscipline, truancy, running away from home, etc. From the end of the 1970s for the entirety of the next decade, the administrative sector continuously contracted, not least under the pressure of the anti-institutional culture of those years, and the referral to re-educative institutions of the 'irregular in conduct and character' had been to all intents and purposes discontinued. Law 616, in delegating the power to implement civil and administrative measures (decided by the juvenile court) to the local authorities, has paradoxically revitalised this sector: the failure to repeal the laws relating to 'irregularity', combined with the scarcity of resources available to many local authorities, has on one hand relegitimised the existence of 're-educative–corrective' measures and on the other has led, in some cases, to the re-use of ex-re-educative institutions as generic institutions for juveniles under administrative and civil measures (in situations of family deprivation, abandonment, etc.)

It is useful to say something, at this point, concerning the decline in the so-called treatment ideology, an ideology which inspired the legal reforms in juvenile justice in 1956, but more generally a *leit-motif*, not only in Italy, for a certain phase in the politics of social control (De Leo 1981; De Leo, Cuomo 1983).

The image of juvenile deviants as 'led astray' – hence morally corrupted, dragged into wrongdoing due to the absence of the capacity for discernment and self-control characteristic of the adult – which is part of an ideology of intervention in terms of 'correction', was a vision dominant during the fascist period. It was succeeded, in changed socio-political conditions and thanks to the late introduction of models and practices from abroad, by a model based on the idea of deprivation and of juvenile delinquency as 'maladjustment'. This model is a therapeutic and indivi-dualising one. Maladjustment, of which offending is seen as a symptom, may indeed have social roots, but manifests itself, and has to be dealt with, on the individual level by means of a series of measures oriented to 're-education' based on the principle of the 'needs' and the 'deficits' of the individual deviant. Offending becomes, and has to be dealt with as, a symptom of individual pathology.

This model inspired, or rather legitimated, the policies of social control, during the 1950s and the early 1960s, in countries with developed welfare states. In Italy, it did not make much inroad as far as adults were concerned (an updated and properly contradictory version emerged in this area only in the penal reforms of 1975), while its adoption in the juvenile area was facilitated by the specific character of juvenile justice (paternalistic, discre-tional, oriented to the 'welfare' of children rather than to their punishment). In this guise it served to provide a 'scientific' substitute for the dated ideology of correction.

But, while in the developed welfare states this model was based on and expressed the common sense of what was by now an extensive network of social services and specialised agencies, both within and outside the criminal justice system, (for the United States see Krisberg, Austin 1978; Empey L.T. 1978, 1979), in Italy it had no other reference points except the traditional ones, entirely internal to the criminal justice system itself. The legitimating ideologies therefore were similar, but the policies and prac-tices of social control in relation to juveniles were quite different.

Apart from a brief flowering of enthusiasm for the already existing re-educative institutions between the end of the 1950s and the beginning of the 1960s, the re-educative ideology only resulted in a change in legitimation for institutions and measures already in operation (Bandini, Gatti 1987). Changes which contributed, nevertheless, to an increase in the sense of frustration and impotence on the part of the professionals and which led to a rapid crisis of this ideology itself. This crisis, paradoxically, often borrowed the language with which it, contemporaneously, was articulated in countries where policies of 're-education' had been concretised in the form of resources and institutions, and where therefore that crisis could not be imputed only to a lack of implementation.

The wave of anti-institutional cultures of the 1970s challenged both the old institutions and the new ideology: the old institutions and the new ideology had not simply failed, rather they had been inspired by mistaken objectives. What was subjected to critique was precisely re-education, criticised because it was a recuperative intervention oriented to the single individual, in accord- ance with a therapeutic model which, by emphasising individual needs and shortcomings, served to legitimate and increase discretionality.

The objective of re-education was succeeded by, or more often, was accompanied during the following years by, the objective of prevention, seen as intervention in and on the social – the community. This objective also had its analogies in other countries (community care, community social work, see Cohen 1985), but the Italian situation is again very specific, both on the political and ideological levels and on that of the resources which were galvanised and which were available.

From 1975 until today, the introduction of new legislative measures has significantly influenced the forms of intervention by juvenile courts. We have said that law 616 of 1977 delegates the implementation of civil and administrative measures decided by the courts to the local authorities. But the reluctance on the part of the judges to make use of administrative measures preceded the passing of the law and can be understood as indicative both of a widespread distrust of the role of closed institutions in performing re-educative tasks and of a re-interpretation of the significance of re-education itself. It was a reluctance which reflected the culture of the early 1970s which deplored the conditions of life in closed institutions (Franchini, Introna 1972; Senzani 1970), at the same time as it criticised their role as mere containers of social problems whose solution should rather be attempted where they are produced: within the community.

There have been and there are various ways of interpreting the issues which this culture considered important. The difference in policies depends on the resources effectively available and mobilisable in the community, and more generally on political and institutional factors rather than being the outcomes of different cultural and political orientations. Indeed, these last may turn out to be *a posteriori* legitimations of institutional and resource constraints.

Overall, two tendencies are identifiable: the first understands the decline of the closed institution in terms of the necessity to deal with the individual case within its own context; the second is characterised by a decisive shift of emphasis on the context, which becomes the primary object of intervention, while the individual problematic situation is left in the background. The first tendency was largely visible in the years preceding the enactment of law 616, due probably to the fact that the responsibility both for the decisions and for their implementation was located exclusively in a central body, the juvenile court, which worked through its own social service agency and whose task was precisely that of handling those individual cases which came to its attention as and when they were defined as problematic. The social context within which the individual case emerged assumed the status of cause of the problem, but it was the problem itself, the individual case, which retained centrality, because it was for this that the court had the entire responsibility.

With the passing of the implementation of administrative measures to the local authorities, the individual problematic case came to be assumed and thereby to disappear within a general category of universalistic welfare and health tasks. Certainly, there are important differences in the ways in which different local authorities have interpreted these tasks (see Bergonzini, Pavarini 1985). But the conflict which often inheres in the relations between courts and local authorities has to do with this point and is in turn reflected in a more general unease expressed culturally as the contrast between explicit demands of social control and welfare tasks. This conflict is acted out on the terrain of policy choices which, in contradictory and fragmented ways, have claimed social and health services as services for all, as responses to *social rights*.

The first result of this situation seems to have been a general resistance on the part of local governments and welfare agencies in the community to the assumption of an explicit social control responsibility. Resistance by such agencies, often justified by reference to universalistic goals and by an approach to problem-solving which privileges the general improvement of the areas under their jurisdiction, risks resulting in the neglect of individual cases, particularly where it combines with the poverty of resources and political and bureaucratic rigidity.

There follows from this a strong push towards the specialisation of interventions and competences: the court assumes the role of an agency among others, to which are attributed mainly tasks of social control. This specialisation does not contribute (as, in principle, it could) to a co-ordinated assumption of responsibility for social problems: rather it produces fragmentation and abandonment. In their turn, fragmentation and abandonment risk leading to the reinforcement of demands for new forms of custodial intervention or for more rigid forms of social control.

THE CONFLICTUAL RELATIONSHIP BETWEEN JUVENILE COURTS AND WELFARE AGENCIES

The present status of juvenile justice appears as particularly contradictory. The processes described above would seem to confine the competence of the juvenile courts to questions of control and intervention exclusively in the area of criminal offending. The issues of deprivation, need, educational and family problems etc., are being removed from the responsibility of courts, though not so much by the law – which upholds the responsibility of the courts in such matters – as by the structure of relations with social services which have a responsibility for these problems at a local level. Juvenile justice shifts decisively towards its tasks of controlling criminally defined behaviours, though of course these tasks are legitimated and organised in a different way to that of adult courts.

It is precisely this difference which is the object of debate and argument. Pressures towards less ambiguous punitive interventions purged of re-educative pretensions, in the name of a less paternalistic and discretional justice, more concerned with 'due process', or in the name of social defence, cohabit with demands for the conservation of the particular characteristics of juvenile justice as the prioritisation of care and protection. The delegation to local authorities of competence in matters of welfare, and juvenile justice's tendential re-shaping of itself as an agency primarily concerned with functions of control, render this debate relevant with respect to the general questions regarding the relationship between criminal justice and the social welfare system. The themes which lie behind them are those relating to the relationship between the social sciences and criminal law.

These issues come to light in particular in the debate around the two types of sentences most frequently pronounced by (Italian) courts in relation to juveniles accused of crime: judicial pardon and acquittal on the grounds of 'immaturity'. Both are judgements which exclude punishment; in the first case because the judge pardons the juvenile judged guilty of the crime ascribed to him/her, in the second case because the juvenile is declared not responsible.

Judicial pardon implies a judgement of guilt, the recognition of criminal responsibility on the part of the juvenile, and expresses the waiver of punishment, on the basis of a favourable prognosis of future behaviour. Legally it is a form of clemency which can be conceded once only, on the first offence. In fact its use is extensive, due to the wide interpretation of this norm by the Constitutional Court (Vaccaro 1982). Today about 40 per cent of criminal proceedings against juveniles (and 57 per cent of all acquittals) end in a pardon.

This is a measure which clearly exemplifies the type of logic which inspires juvenile justice: the waiver of punishment should be based in fact on an evaluation of the personality of the juvenile and of the social and cultural circumstances within which the offence was situated, such as to indicate a 'repentance' on the part of the juvenile him or herself. With the pardon juvenile justice acts paternalistically: 'You have done wrong, but this time, and on the basis of a promise that you will not do it again, I will forgo punishing you.' In reality judicial practice has given pardon quite a different significance: it is indicative of a tendency towards a *de facto* depenalisation. Conceded usually ritually, at the end of the preliminary hearing or *in camera*, without there having been any direct rapport between the judge and the juvenile, it is a measure which is by now an automatic obligation rather than a benefit conceded in the light of particular consider- ations relating to a particular individual: it assumes the bureaucratic and impersonal characteristics of an amnesty. Purged of 're-educative' ambitions, conceded in general without there having been, as the law would still imply,[6] any specific evaluation of the likelihood of 'repentance', the pardon expresses nowadays an implicitly negative evaluation of the laws and procedures by means of which the case is brought to court.

This use of the pardon can be read as an indication of that division of tasks among agencies of which we have spoken. It indicates, in fact, an implicit renunciation by the court of its re-educative tasks. If deemed appropriate, the judge will open administrative proceedings, delegating *de facto* these tasks to the local authorities. Alternatively, s/he will give a security order: but the relevant considerations will not be, in this case, of a re-educative nature but rather of social defence.

It is precisely this tendency which is criticised and sharply contested by some members of the judiciary (Vaccaro 1982) for whom the pardon should retain its original significance of an individual favour to be conceded on the basis of a 'considered prognostic evaluation', within a meaningful relationship between judge and juvenile, in which the con- cession of the pardon takes the form of an instrument to achieve 'repent- ance'. The exercise of the power to punish, according to these judges, has to be bent, in the case of juveniles, towards re-educative ends of which the judge him/herself should continue to be the principal interpreter and prota- gonist, at once severe and paternal. In this conception the juvenile judge reassumes the competences and knowledges which traditionally make reference to the father figure but which today are, by contrast, the prero- gative of a multiplicity of 'experts': educationalists, psychologists, socio- logists, social workers, psychiatrists, doctors, etc. The judge can of course, though it is not obligatory, make use of this expertise. The new code of criminal procedure in juvenile cases, if on the one hand it shifts the focus of 'expert' investigations from the personality of the juvenile towards the personal, family, social conditions and resources, on the other hand it further extends the discretional power of the judge, confirming juvenile justice in its difference and separateness. Of this more later.

The debate around the judgement of the non-liability of juveniles by reason of 'immaturity' – a verdict of acquittal less frequent than pardon, and nevertheless widely utilised (the rate of use varies between courts, see AA.VV 1982, indicating not so much a geographical variability of the levels of immaturity of juveniles, as different cultures of judges: but also different social, political and institutional conditions)[7] presents some analogies with the debate on the non-liability of the mentally ill by reason of 'incapacity of understanding and intention'.[8]

By contrast with mental disability, immaturity is a transitory, non pathological condition and specific to juveniles. What it refers to, from the strictly legal point of view, is already, however, a controversial question. The norm (article 98 of the penal code) prescribes that for juveniles between fourteen and eighteen years (under fourteens are never criminally responsible) the capacity of 'understanding and intention' cannot be presumed, and has to be ascertained in each case. Because it is a question of a capacity linked to age, interpretative divergencies already arise in relation to the parameters of comparison. Is a boy who has reached the level of 'normal maturation' for his age group capable of understanding and intention? In this case and for the same criminal act, seventeen year olds could be declared non-liable while fourteen year olds are liable? Or should the standard of normality be represented by an eighteen year old? (male? female?) The two interpretations have evidently very different consequences for the extent of the area of liability (see Barsotti *et al.* 1976; Vercellone 1982).

Even more than in the case of pardon, which new legal proposals would extend to adults (not by chance within a paternalistic-repressive ideology, and for transgressions of the law that oscillate between 'vice' and sickness and for 'private' transgressions, on principle without victims – as with the proposed bill on drug addiction), the acquittal by reason of immaturity characterises juvenile justice as different, insofar as juveniles and especially, it seems, girls (as it is girls who are more often acquitted by reason of immaturity, see Faccioli, Pitch 1988) are different physiologically and psychologically, from adults. It is a difference clearly identified as deficiency, which encourages the production of scientific, psychological and sociological theories to justify it and give it content. However much it is used in a 'bureaucratic' mode, unaccompanied by procedures and expert assessments and in the role purely of a justification for acquittal, the judgement of immaturity arouses a level of annoyance and concern among judges that pardon does not, precisely because of its specificity and its reference to knowledges and competences, which many judges today pronounce as outside their sphere of competence.

In the case of the capacity for understanding and intention on the part of adults, the body of knowledge referred to is exclusively psychiatry, since for adults incapacity is based on a hypothesis of mental illness. In the case of juveniles, the capacity of understanding and intention is connected to something still more uncertain and undefined, if that were possible, than mental illness. What can be meant by 'maturity'? What bodies of knowledge are authorised to evaluate it? As in the case of incapacity due to infirmity of mind, so also in the case of immaturity, developments in, and the crisis of, psychiatric and psychological knowledge have given rise to debates in which the scientific status of categories like immaturity and incapacity and the possibility of establishing linear relations between one and the other, have come under increasing criticism (see Cuomo, La Greca, Viggiani 1982).

The boundaries between criminal law and the social sciences become, again, the object of conflict and discussion resulting in a complex situation of institutional uncertainty in which the tendency to separate spheres of competence renders problematic the assumption of responsibility on the part of the different actors involved.

Among judges two main positions can be identified. On one hand are those who, with various shades of opinion and appealing to a variety of imperatives, tend to emphasise the tendency to separation of competences and redefine the proper tasks of the judiciary in a restrictive mode which excludes a re-educative function. On the other hand, there are those judges who respond to institutional uncertainty by extending their competences and responsibilities: assuming as internal to their own function an evaluation of immaturity involving not only a diagnosis of the personality of the juvenile at a psychological level, but also analyses which take into consideration the social and cultural context.

Where the first group denounces ambiguity, uncertainty and discretion both in respect of the use of the verdict, and of its effects,[9] the second group, in defending a measure which takes adequate account of the particular status (in the psychological sense) of individuals 'still in the process of formation', demands that juvenile justice retains its traditional role of guardian of the welfare of the juvenile, and confirms that its tasks are different to those of ordinary justice (Vaccaro 1982a).

Acquittal on grounds of immaturity, for this latter group of judges, does not have to be, as it is now, like pardon, a more or less bureaucratic form of depenalisation, but can become – or rather return to being – the result of a complex investigation of which the protagonist is the judge. These judges seek to dissociate themselves from the uncertainty of psychiatric and psychological diagnoses – which other judges and psychologists denounce as untrustworthy and incompatible with the language and goals of law (Dusi 1982; Forato 1982) – and anchor immaturity in the social and cultural characteristics of the life of the juvenile.

'Immature' is in this case the juvenile who is socially, culturally, economically underprivileged. The investigation of these conditions can indeed be entrusted to experts, but it remains to the judge to assume the responsibility for their evaluation and for deciding whether they constitute a situation of sufficient deprivation as to justify acquittal. Immaturity becomes here a socio-political diagnosis: the judge, aware of the selectivity of justice, decides to overturn its direction. 'Privileged' juveniles will be punished, others not.

The debate on the two main types of acquittal, and above all the discussion of the problem of immaturity, signals the intensification of reflection among juvenile court judges about their proper tasks and responsibilities and the changing of their professional standards in the context of the institutional uncertainty which we have noted.

It is an uncertainty which presents many faces: the absorption of the welfare and protection tasks of juvenile justice into the universe of social rights has involved, among other things, the increasing separation between the aims of control directed to social defence, and those directed to welfare and protection; it is a separation pertaining as much to the institutions as to the culture of the professionals and is to be seen within the more general dynamics of control policies.

If present policies (see chapter 1) seem pervaded by a double and contradictory logic – on the one hand decarceration, de-institutionalisation, and on the other reinforced control in the community, new criminalisations performing a symbolic function (see the law on prison reform 616, 1986; the new law re-criminalising drug use; the new code of juvenile court procedure; many of the proposals to modify the psychiatric reform law) – they nevertheless seek legitimation through a discourse which both articulates the common sense of the welfare state and that of its crisis, and which at the same time offers an explanation of this crisis: that which cannot be cured, actually refuses treatment or is incurable.

In the first case there is a wilful resistance which requires a criminalising response, or recourse to the symbolic potential of criminal law: as is presently the case with drug dependency. This also means that the status of illness and need at the basis of the culture of the medical and social services, not only does not cancel, for the professionals as much as for the clients, attributions and assumptions of responsibility, but also becomes fragile and ambiguous in times of crisis. Criminalisation is then invoked as an instrument with which to motivate the healthy, conscious part of the drug-dependent to treat that which however remains constructed prevalently as illness. The continuity between (threat of) imprisonment and community care becomes explicit.

In the second case, resistance to treatment is not intentional, but precisely because of this, is a danger to society. The response, again, involves institutionalisation. Such a response informs many proposals to modify the Italian law on psychiatric reform.

In both cases cure and care explicitly take on connotations of social control oriented to repression and social defence. Yet, the public social services, and many private ones, continue to reject these tasks.[10]

The case of juveniles is somehow paradoxical. There is no doubt that, in Italy, if we go by the criminal statistics, there is not a real problem of juvenile delinquency. In fact, the percentage of juveniles sentenced is so low that it ought to encourage a vigorous process of depenalisation,[11] and the rejection of any form of imprisonment. The difference and separateness of juvenile justice, with the resulting ambiguity, discretionality, attenuation of judicial safeguards, has hitherto permitted and legitimated a very limited exercise of the penal sanction. However, the ambiguous nature of the rejection of imprisonment, the resistance to the development of a policy of depenalisation, together with the coexistence of re-educative and welfare aspects make juvenile justice vulnerable to oscillations in response to changes in the prevailing climate of social control and social defence.

The unease of juvenile court judges must be understood within this social and political context and the various solutions advanced to deal with it must be analysed as attempts to redefine the judges' own professional identity, but they also must be evaluated with respect to the consequences they might involve. I will examine the latter for convenience under two aspects: the 'internal' aspect defined as the tasks of juvenile justice in relation to juveniles themselves; and the 'external' aspect, defined as the tasks of juvenile justice in relation to society.

A JUSTICE OF RIGHTS VS. A JUSTICE OF NEEDS: A FALSE DILEMMA?

The two tendencies which emerge in the debate on judicial pardon and immaturity both place themselves within a 'liberal' orientation, whose key elements are depenalisation and decarceration, and which is explicitly critical of the repressive and punitive functions of criminal justice. They are however different in logic and consequences. The first takes the road of a new formalism while in the second the substantivist position is confirmed and reinforced.

The first, restrictive, orientation emphasises the centrality of the rights of juveniles, namely liberty rights. These are seen as undermined by the preoccupation with re-education embraced by a justice based on needs, which is accused of a discretionality and a paternalism conducive to oppressive results. The second tendency insists on the priority of the needs of juveniles, while seeing in a justice of rights the risks of formalism, rigidity, purely retributionist effects.

Both tendencies justify themselves through an appeal to the 'good' of the juvenile: so that even the first position, formalist and potentially retributionist as far as procedures and solutions to adopt, entrusts to them a pedagogic function.

The arguments relating to the verdict of acquittal on grounds of immaturity are significant summaries of the two positions. For judges oriented towards a justice of needs, immaturity is understood as a *condition* resulting from the interaction of a variety of processes: familial, environmental, social. But the criminal justice system's influence on this condition is not seen as part of these processes. The model underlining this position is characterised by a determinism in which 'deviance' is conceived as the effect of certain specific types of deficiencies. Whether these deficiencies are to be identified on the level of the social, rather than the biological or psychological, certainly changes the type of intervention, but not the basic determinism itself to which end even the interactionist contribution of labelling theory is bent: social and penal stigmatisations are treated as causes. Immaturity is seen as a characteristic of the subject – diagnosed by judges and used as the rationale for their judgements – which is the basis and 'cause' of the delinquent act. The diagnosis of immaturity – for those judges who want to recover its full significance, rescuing it from its present 'merely bureaucratic' use, in its acquittal function – opens up the possibility of adopting measures of protection justified in terms of deficiencies and needs.

These measures, apart from that of security, which is given on the basis of the 'social dangerousness' of the individual, non-liable because immature, are not, following the virtual abolition of re-educative institutions, very different from those which judges can dispose for any juvenile judged in a condition of need, before, after, or independently of a criminal sentence: the intervention of the social worker, the prescription of particular obligations of work or study, the referral to a therapeutic community, etc. Though the adoptable measures are the same, nevertheless this approach to the problem of immaturity confers, in principle, extensive powers on juvenile judges, confirming their dominant role in relation to that of social work. In a context of malfunctioning social services, for whatever reason, and in political situations characterised by plans to reduce welfare expenditures, a position of this type can be useful both on the ideological and on the practical level to support aspects of the welfare system itself. The risks, on the other hand, follow from the wide discretion conferred on the juvenile judge, especially in a system, such as ours, which retains the recourse to security measures, as a substitute for, or in addition to penal sanctions.

The new Italian code of juvenile penal procedure is imbued with a logic very similar to that described above: where the possibilities of acquittal are extended (quashing of an indictment because of 'lack of evidence and intent', or when normal proceedings would be 'prejudicial to the educative needs of the juvenile'), and the possibilities of decarceration (conditional discharge, attendance orders, supervision orders) are also multiplied, this code extends the discretionary power of the judge, and confirms and reinforces his/her competence to decide the liability and degree of responsibility of the accused (no longer based on an evaluation of the 'personality' of the juvenile, but through 'the acquisition of elements concerning personal, family, social and environmental conditions and resources'), and makes available, in cases of acquittal, or in addition to a penal sanction, a series of security measures (probation, house arrest, court order for work or study) which could extend the scope of intervention and the size of the population vulnerable to such interventions. There is also the security measure applicable to those, non-liable but declared dangerous, who have committed offences for which the punishment is not less than twelve years: juvenile custody is substituted by 'treatment in the community'. The result is the *de facto* assigning of tasks of social defence to welfare agencies, many of which are private: with the possible consequences both of exporting the prison model into the 'community' (see Pavarini 1986) and of its privatisation.

In a justice oriented to rights, the proposal to abolish non-liability by reason of immaturity would be established on the basis of an understanding of responsibility similar to that which we shall analyse in relation to the liability of the mentally disabled. The judgement of immaturity is considered here as itself productive of immaturity, that is as depriving the subject of sense, consciousness and control over her/his own actions. Immaturity is understood not as a condition, but as the possible result of processes among which is included the relationship with criminal justice. In this reading 'responsibility' is identified not as a property of the subject, but rather as a complex link between subject and action, within a specific cultural context on the basis of whose values and norms those links are interpreted, and productive of 'practical and symbolic effects' which act and react on the links themselves (De Leo 1985). Responsibility, criminal responsibility and liability are here assimilated: an assimilation made possible by the rediscovery that sociological and psychological theory and classical theory of law utilise the same model to distinguish action from behaviour. At the centre of this distinction is precisely the category of responsibility (De Giorgi 1984; Giddens 1979).

The recognition of liability becomes, in this reading, itself potentially productive of consciousness through triggering off a process of assumption of responsibility (in this case, on the part of juveniles). On the practical level, this implies that the judicial response be based on the actions of offenders rather than on the evaluation of their personality: which would imply the abolition of security measures and of the administrative competences of the court. The question of needs, of the particularity of the individual situation, would not be evaded: rather a specificity based on the characteristics of the action would be substituted for one based on the characteristics of the actor, in relation to the type of link between the authority responsible for intervention and the juvenile responsible for the action, and with regard to the level of 'acceptance of responsibility expressed by the juvenile' (see De Leo 1985)

This is actually a position which seeks to overcome the polarisation between a merely retributivist justice oriented to rights and a justice oriented to needs. A justice which, in opposition to formalism, is based on a non-reductionist concept of rights, and in opposition to substantivism, seeks to transform needs into social rights. The conflict over the distribution of responsibility between court and welfare agencies would be overcome in a model of co-ordinated intervention for which the court should function as external guarantor.

As to the redefinition of the professional identity of the judge, the position under discussion here proposes not a multi-expert judge exercising hegemony over social work expertise, but a judging judge, supreme guarantor of the rights of the juvenile: yet nevertheless, in some respects contradictorily, both pedagogue and re-educator precisely in carrying out his legal tasks.

There are in fact at least two problems which leave this proposal open to risky, or at least ambiguous, consequences.

The first refers precisely to the equivalence established between responsibility, criminal responsibility and liability, or between the indictment proceedings which take place in a court room and the processes of social responsibilisation. These equivalences are to be questioned not only with respect to their 'scientific' correctness, but also with regard to the logic they embody and their possible practical consequences. Such equivalence confers on the penal sanction a specific utility: that of rendering the convicted offender 'responsible'; which means however that, if the penal response is given to the action it retains the function of changing the 'personality' of the subject. The penal response is thus 'good' for the person sentenced: should it thus function as the equivalent of, or substitute for, a type of therapy or moral pedagogy?

The other question left open is that of security and social defence. In fact, if, in principle, this proposal is located in a model which identifies the functions of social control as unavoidable and fundamental, both as regards criminal justice and other agencies (family, school, social services), it does not take adequate account of the fact that only the criminal justice system is competent, not simply to impose sanctions (something which however occurs in different forms within these other agencies), but to impose them by force. Social institutions and the welfare system are productive of social control (and one can think of ways by which this production can be explicit and non-injurious to the liberty rights of the individual subject): but such control can only be the result of an interaction in which the subject freely participates. Otherwise, the carcerial model risks being exported again outside the penal system.

The problem of the relationship between coercion and consent is not resolved by delegating coercion to the sphere of penal intervention: it is present also in the welfare system and it is here that it has to be confronted if a further expansion of the penal sanction, seeking new legitimacy in terms of 'due process', 'inculcation of responsibility', and rediscovery of the pedagogic function of punishment, is to be avoided. It is certainly not difficult to think of a scenario in which moral panic campaigns focused on 'danger' lead to a re-enlargement of the role of the penal and where moral panics focused on deprivation lead to a coercive form of welfare.[12]

WHOSE RESPONSIBILITY?

The complex relations between criminal justice and social welfare systems constitute, as has been said, a circular process, the results of which, besides the production of chronicity, may be abandonment, and its correlate, social dangerousness. The present situation in Italy appears very different from that described for example in the United States or Great Britain (see Faccioli 1988) – at present in Italy the risk of an extension of the network of control through the welfare institutions is non-existent. The welfare state is smaller, particularly in the areas concerned with juveniles in trouble. Yet it is a situation characterised by such institutional uncertainty, confusion of boundaries, shifting of responsibilities that it might result in a growth in social deprivation and dangerousness: where deprivation becomes represented as an unmanageable problem it assumes the form of disturbance or dangerousness.[13] At present, therefore, although 'delinquency' is not regarded as a serious social problem, its growth remains a possibility as the area of deprivation and consequentially social dangerousness grows. Such a growth, and the way in which it comes to be perceived – precisely as deprivation or delinquency, a problem of the agencies of social control or a problem of the individuals – depends on the relations and conflicts between agencies, and these themselves change in relation not only to the politics of legislation, and the ideologies which legitimise them, but also in relation to the resources at their disposal, their mode of utilisation and the outcome of the continuous negotiations and conflicts between agencies and users.

The question of responsibility must then be posed well outside the boundaries defined by criminal responsibility and liability. It must be constructed as a problem relating to the reciprocal tasks assigned and discharged by juvenile justice, local government, the school, the family. Thus displaced, the responsibility of the individual juvenile may be reconceptualised. Those concerned with the juvenile's rights wish to reconstruct her status as that of the independent actor of adult justice; those concerned with the juvenile's needs stress her present status of dependency. The first view the presumption of autonomy as either an indispensable principle of criminal justice or (contradictorily, as we have seen) as a means to induce autonomy itself. The second see autonomy as diminished by what makes a juvenile a juvenile: her age, her being economically dependent, her still being in a process of educational formation, etc. But, if we locate the search for responsibility in the interplay of the different agencies that are supposed to care for the juvenile, then her own responsibility might be looked for in the relationships she establishes with these agencies: independence as a function, rather than the opposite, of dependence. And if we decide that we prefer to limit as far as possible recourse not only to incarceration proper, but also to any other form of segregation, custody, isolation or comprehensive care, the central responsibility on the part of the professionals and above all the judiciary, becomes – besides that of minimising the production of deprivation – the conscious assumption of the risk of producing social insecurity: the task, that is, of broadening and extending the limits of compatibility and tolerance of the social system.

6 Criminal responsibility and mental illness

The criminal justice system and the new psychiatry

Another area rich in examples of the relationship between the discourse of criminal law and that of the social sciences – and between the practices of the criminal justice system and those of social work and welfare – is to be found at the interface of psychiatry and criminal justice.

This has always been a field of uncertain definitions, riven with tensions and conflicts (see for example, Foucault 1976; Georget 1984). Yet such tensions are all the more visible today, when the innovations in psychiatric concepts and practices (in Italy sanctioned by the reform law 180 of 1978, and now integrated in law 833 on health reform), have put into question the traditional equilibrium between the two systems both on the theoretical and practical levels.

These developments have given rise to an institutional uncertainty within which innovations, attempts at adjustment, re-elaborations and revisions have taken place. The main actors in this process are criminal justice professionals, forensic psychiatrists, judges, psychiatric workers, associations of relatives of mentally disabled, and other voluntary groups. It is a rich and shifting scenario, of which here I will only explore a few aspects, on the basis of a research project which looked at the Milan criminal court between 1984 and 1987.[1]

THEORETICAL AND POLICY QUESTIONS

The innovations, over the last thirty years, in the theory, practice, and legal status of Italian psychiatry have transformed the context in which the following questions are posed: the criminal responsibility and the social dangerousness of the criminally mentally disabled; the tasks and therefore the responsibilities of criminal justice professionals, forensic psychiatrists, and the workers in the new community based mental health services. Although analogous innovations have occurred in all Western countries during the last thirty years the developments in Italy have been the most coherent and radical (for a more detailed analysis, see De Leonardis 1988a).[2]

The crisis of a psychiatry based around the dual concept of treatment–custody has resulted in the emergence of a plurality of approaches, often in competition or conflict among themselves. It has, moreover, contributed to the destabilisation of the traditional pact between psychiatry and criminal justice. This pact involved psychiatry, as the handmaid of law (Betti, Pavarini 1984; Manacorda 1982), in providing the criminal justice system, on the one hand with a scientific legitimation for cases of exclusion from punishment (unfitness to plead, etc.) and on the other with a causal connection between mental disability and social dangerousness which served as justification for the system of security measures (prison asylum, institutions of care and custody) for the so-called criminally insane. At the same time psychiatric institutions took charge of the custodial control of a heterogeneous population whose problems overflowed the scientific and professional boundaries of other institutions (like medicine and criminal justice) to provide what De Leonardis has appropriately characterised as the administration of an 'institutional residue'.

This pact has fallen irredeemably into crisis. Whatever the directions taken by the theories and practices of psychiatry during the last thirty years, what has ceased to exist is that particular interfacing of care and custody which characterised the asylum as an institution and psychiatry as the body of knowledge constructed around 'insanity'. Whether psychiatry currently rejects its mandate of social control in favour of a redefinition in more strictly medical terms or whether such a mandate is undergoing critical re-elaboration as an aspect of proper therapeutic competence, it has by now formed part of that complex of knowledges, disciplines and practices which help define the sphere of social citizenship. The civilising of psychiatry, confirmed in Italy by the reforms of 1978, has inserted it as a component of the structure of social rights. As an aspect of health reform, psychiatry becomes a service regulated by the principles of the right to health which the reform recognises and sanctions.

But the crisis of asylum psychiatry has also resulted in a revision of the theoretical status of mental illness and to a questioning of diagnostic categories such as to render their deployment in the criminal justice field uncertain and problematic. This has occurred above all with respect to the connection between mental illness and fitness to plead (for an acute analysis of this matter from the standpoint of jurisprudence see Bertolino 1988).

Even in this area different tendencies co-exist, and it is characteristic of the current period that no tendency can today claim to be hegemonic, a fact which of itself contributes to the production of an area of uncertainty in relations with criminal justice, the latter demanding 'scientifically' un-ambiguous and uncontested definitions.

But, furthermore, not only is there no agreement among the different tendencies on how to define and classify mental illness; there is also a generalised retreat from diagnosis, or rather the preference, consistent with the shifting of emphasis on psychiatry's therapeutic vocation, to deal with the individual rather than the illness. The dissolution of the causal link: mental illness – lack of free will, is a consequence. Today there are few psychiatrists who would allow themselves to affirm that a particular mental problem, however diagnosed, is, in itself, the cause of an absence of consciousness and control over the individual's own actions. The category of free will and the capacity or incapacity to act in accordance with will and intention,[3] is largely considered as meaningless from a psychiatric point of view, in the same way as that of immaturity in the case of juveniles, and thus fitness to plead becomes a juridical category on which psychiatry can neither confer a scientific status nor provide empirical content.

There are, moreover, aspects of the therapeutic orientation of contem-porary psychiatry which bring it directly into conflict with the demands and exigencies of criminal justice. To take one example, the idea is increasingly making headway in advanced psychiatric thinking that the attempt to ascertain the capacity or incapacity of an individual for intentional action is impossible. I have already noted this with regard to juveniles. Social psychology and the most progressive areas of psychiatry are in agreement both in considering 'responsibility' the result of an interactive process (as with the theory of attribution) rather than an individual quality which either is or is not, and in considering this process as indispensable to the thera-peutic project.[4]

The Italian law on psychiatric reform, which abolished compulsory institutionalisation and established the closure of psychiatric hospitals, not only confirmed treatment as a social right, but also determined that it can only be given outside custody, through a local network of mental health services integrated into the national health service. This implies the delegi-timation of the security measure of confinement to penal psychiatric hospitals for the 'treatment and custody' of defendants judged unfit to plead because of insanity and who are declared to be socially dangerous (on the question of penal psychiatric hospitals see Manacorda 1982, 1988; Daga 1985).[5]

Before discussing the question of social dangerousness, I would like to underline again how the Italian psychiatric reform creates a situation radically different, on the levels of professional culture and practice, from that which has occurred in other countries also involved in processes of de-institutionalisation. The abolition of psychiatric hospitals renders it in principle impossible on the part of the social services and the criminal justice system to refer a 'hard core' of persons and problems to a separate specialised institution. This implies that the social services have to take charge of all kinds of psychiatric disturbances, however manifested. The legislation aimed at a clear contrast with the tendencies evident in other countries towards the creation of a 'circuit' of psychiatric institutions working through the processes of selection and referral. The law aimed to avoid what has been called the 'psychiatrisation' of the community, i.e. an extension of soft psychiatric control which does not substitute but on the contrary requires and needs 'hard', closed, psychiatric 'sites' delegated to take charge of those problems and individuals previously handled by the old asylum.[6]

As will be seen, the psychiatric services have interpreted, and continue to interpret, this mandate in various ways, not only in relation to the prevalence of differing conceptions of psychiatry, but also as a result of organisational constraints, availability of resources, and, not least, the attitudes and behaviour of other institutions, political, medical, welfare and police. Nevertheless, the lack, at least in principle, of a clear and separate space for a 'hard core' within the network of psychiatric services, complicates even more the interaction between the latter and the criminal justice system. That grey area at the boundary between social disturbance and psychiatric disorder traditionally lying within the competence of the asylum, is today the object of redefinition and debate – both institutionally and at the level of political and social conflicts. On the other hand, the urgent problem posed by the existence of penal psychiatric hospitals merges with that of the non-existence of separate and 'secure' non-penal psychiatric institutions.

In addition, the social dangerousness of the mentally ill, now that it cannot be presumed even from the legal standpoint (in 1982 with the judgement of the Constitutional Court; in 1986 with the law on prison reform – the Gozzini law) but has to be ascertained for each individual case, has become a question which psychiatrists, both clinical and forensic, agree on seeing as outside their professional competence.[7]

The question has two aspects. The first has to do with the traditional assumption of the existence of a connection between mental illness and the propensity to commit criminal acts. Much research has established the non-existence of such a connection. Mentally disturbed people commit no more crimes generally than the population as a whole. Neither do they commit a disproportionate number of crimes involving violence to property or persons. The second aspect is concerned with the ability of psychiatry to predict the future behaviour of mentally ill offenders. Again, research has established that, from a psychiatric point of view, such prediction is impossible. On the other hand, as in the case of capacity for intentional action, the category of social dangerousness is rejected as lacking meaning and scientific content. It has an exclusively juridical significance, and many commentators (see the review in Traverso 1979) have noted how psychiatrists have a tendency to engage in hyper-prediction, as a result of pressure from the judiciary and the preoccupation of the latter with matters of social defence (see also Bandini, Gatti 1982; 1985).

This brings us to the problem of the present status of forensic psychiatry, i.e. of that area of psychiatry traditionally concerned with deciding upon the capacity or otherwise of defendants to engage in intentional action and upon the social dangerousness of those defendants suspected of mental disability through the instrument of the psychiatric report. It has already been noted that such a role is based on a double loyalty: on one hand to the standards of psychiatry and on the other to the exigencies of the criminal justice system. This 'duplicity' could remain implicit and invisible, and the two sides avoid conflict, as long as the hegemony of asylum psychiatry remained undiminished. But the prevalent treatment orientation together with the general crisis of traditional diagnostic categories, and the abandonment of predictive pretensions regarding social dangerousness has made this conflict today both evident and unavoidable. There is currently a considerable debate on these questions amongst the more thoughtful forensic psychiatrists[8] as part of an attempt to redefine the proper tasks and responsibilities of the discipline.

But the present scenario is characterised by the simultaneous presence of a heterogeneity of actors. Not only forensic psychiatrists but also clinical psychiatrists and in general social service professionals, especially in some local situations, (Trieste and Perugia for example), either despite themselves or through conscious choice, interact – frequently conflictually – with the criminal justice agencies.

Rather than attempt to follow through all aspects of this interaction I will limit myself to a consideration of some of the problems relating to the questions of the fitness to plead and the social dangerousness of the mentally ill defendant. In relation to the criminal justice system I will focus on issues relating to preliminary judicial investigation and trial proceedings.[9] These are both the terminal points of proceedings involving psychiatric and welfare agencies together with the police and law enforcement agencies, and the starting points for proceedings which involve other agencies such as the prison, social services, penal psychiatric hospitals etc.

The innovations described above have 'enlivened', so it has been said, the relations between psychiatry and criminal justice, creating an area of institutional uncertainty which has acted as a fertile area for innovations in various directions. But the criminal justice system also has been subject to notable innovative pressures, both on the 'output' side (prison reform), on the trial level (the reform of the code of criminal procedure), and more generally as regards jurisprudential orientations and investigation procedures. Some of these innovations have been introduced by legislation, others by practice. All aspects and areas of the criminal justice system have been touched by these developments, from the judiciary to police and prison staff. While not claiming to give a full account of the different interpretations of these innovations, I will identify some of the tendencies currently contributing to tension in the relations between criminal justice and psychiatry in particular, and the system of welfare and treatment in general.

On the legislative plane, an important development has been the removal (albeit ambivalent and incomplete) from the criminal justice system of questions such as drug use and, at least in part, juvenile delinquency, and their consignment to the areas of treatment and welfare. This has been accompanied by a tendency to what Pavarini (1986) has called 'hyper-criminalisation' or the development of an administrative criminal law subordinated to political exigencies (on this point see Ferrarese 1984 on the changes in the status and in the function of the judges, and more generally, Resta 1983). The promulgation of emergency legislation in relation to terrorism has been the predominant factor in this area. Another important development has to do with the legislation which has introduced alternatives to custodial punishment, and *de facto* flexibility of penalties into the Italian criminal justice system (the so-called Gozzini law, 1986, see Di Lazzaro 1988; Mosconi 1988; Pavarini 1988), thus instituting official channels for the conduct of relations between the criminal justice system and the local institutions of care and welfare.

On the level of jurisprudence, we may note the affirmation of a substantivist tendency, of a criminal law focusing on the offender rather than the offence, which was undoubtedly reinforced by emergency legislation. However, such a tendency is not understandable exclusively in terms of social defence. Substantivist tendencies with a 'left' orientation were, as already noted, present from the 1970s onwards, as calls to take account of the concrete facts of inequality, individual neglect, etc. This tendency, therefore, on one hand is manifested in the proliferation of 'risk' crimes (see Fiandaca 1984) and in the increasingly confident recourse by the courts to verdicts of social dangerousness (see Robert 1982);[10] on the other hand in a strong focus on the consequences of punishment for the individual offender, in relation to her or his history, social and cultural circumstances etc.

The result is that judges, above all those involved in the investigation proceedings, develop complex relations, even if not always explicit or official, with welfare and voluntary institutions, therapeutic communities etc., and they become not only political but also social actors. This development is legitimated by an ideology of punishment which emphasises rehabilitation, re-education and resocialisation, but also by the introduction of alternatives to custody oriented, at least in principle, to the personality of the offender, rather than the offence committed.

All this re-introduces for criminal justice both specific questions such as that of fitness to plead and social dangerousness of individual defendants, and general issues of competence, conflict, and relationship with other languages, knowledges and practices. The orientation to consequences, typical of a criminal law subordinated to the requirements of general politics, and expressed in a focus on the offender, meets but also clashes with those knowledges, institutions and practices oriented to treatment and welfare. These last both lend support to the criminal justice system, providing it with off-loading points and a scientific legitimation and, at the same time, enter into competition with it, through both demanding greater competences for themselves and by making use of the criminal justice system as a place for the referral of all those problems which fall outside their own operative categories. The metaphor of 'circuit' was used to describe this process in relation to juvenile delinquency. What happens with psychiatry, in relation to that vast grey area in which interaction and blurring takes place between psychiatric problems, poverty, neglect and social disturbance, is largely analogous.[11]

In this context, characterised by fluidity, and normative and institutional uncertainty, it is interesting to see how specific actors, in specific situations, interpret their tasks and take decisions; how scientific paradigms, value positions, competences and powers concretely interact; how local innovations are produced by the conflicts, the negotiations and exchanges between actors, institutions and knowledges (see Donolo, Fichera 1988) and what their effects are on re-articulating the relationships between civil and social rights, between rights and needs. In short, it is interesting to reconstruct the 'institutional daily life' (see De Leonardis *et al.* 1988, Introduction) as experienced and lived by the actors themselves, highlighting the areas of concrete choice activated by them in the context of those legal, organisational and resource constraints in which they find themselves.

It is precisely within these areas open to choice that I shall look for the ways in which responsibility is concretely defined and assumed. And it is through this research strategy that I attempted to reconstruct the heterogeneous dynamic of the distribution of social control, otherwise assumed as having unidirectional, totalitarian and pervasive tendencies.

THE DILEMMA OF FORENSIC PSYCHIATRY: WHO ARE ITS REAL CLIENTS?

The innovations in the penal field and those on the side of clinical psychiatry have both extended and problematised the sphere of competence of forensic psychiatry. More precisely, there is an increase and a diversification of recourse by the criminal justice system to 'expert' opinion. On the other hand, the greater room conceded to bodies of knowledge outside law contributes to an increase in the discretional autonomy of the judge who remains *peritus peritorum*, the sole qualified to decide. The result is a situation in which the increased responsibilities of the judge pushes her to seek comfort and legitimation in external knowledges, through opinions which are 'objectively' motivated, certain, and provide articulate 'explanations'.

Because forensic psychiatry is, at least hitherto, the only body of knowledge external to law authorised to contribute evidence – by means of the *perizia psichiatrica*: a written report based on one or more examinations of the accused, plus oral testimony in court – on the life and the personality of the accused and the psychological circumstances of the crime, it is not surprising that judges make increasing recourse to it, not only when there are strong indications of the presence of mental distress, but also in cases of particularly serious offences, or where the motivations of the offender are not immediately comprehensible.[12]

Psychiatric court reports become overloaded with demands and expectations which help to make their boundaries uncertain and their effects confused at precisely the same time as innovations in clinical psychiatry have resulted in a crisis of the old methodologies and presuppositions and when the very existence and relevance of psychiatric reports is the subject of debates and reforms.[13]

The demands of judges, increasingly seen as ambiguous and inappropriate, for expert 'clarifications' (Luberto, De Fazio 1986); together with the present changes within psychiatry – the diversification of tendencies, accentuation of therapeutic orientations, problematisation not only of traditional diagnostic categories but of the nosological–taxonomic foundation itself – mean that forensic psychiatrists are having to handle wider areas, redefine their professional competences, rethink their relationship with the criminal justice system and seek out new relations with a community based clinical psychiatry.

There are different orientations among forensic psychiatrists but all aim at a recovery of autonomy and specificity in relation both to the criminal justice system and to clinical psychiatry. There are certainly elements of professional opportunism in play but, whatever the motivations, the implications both for criminal justice and community psychiatry are considerable. Professional autonomy is regained (or demanded) precisely on the diagnostic terrain: but it is the methods of diagnoses which are changing and diagnosis itself tends to lose nosological rigidity – and that gives rise to new problems, as will be seen.

It is generally recognised by forensic psychiatrists that the juridical concept of capacity or incapacity for intentional action is meaningless in psychiatric terms. Yet, since this concept is both fundamental for a criminal law embodying due process and at the root of common sense evaluations, the task of forensic psychiatry is seen as that of constructing bridges between the two. The basis for this is a clinical knowledge reinforced by considerations relating to the context, timing and particular form taken by the disturbance in question. Thus the question of incapacity becomes autonomous from, and demands an ulterior investigation with respect to the existence of 'mental illness'. The assessment of incapacity and its eventual relationship with the existence of an 'illness' fall into the field of competence of forensic psychiatry, as opposed to clinical psychiatry. This, in the opinion of many forensic psychiatrists, arises from a fundamental issue of professional ethics. It would be a betrayal of the therapeutic relationship to engage in relations with the patient in which the aim of cure is subordinated to (or in conflict with) diagnostic tasks oriented to establishing liability for punishment; all the more so insofar as clinical psychiatry argues the anti-therapeutic nature of the consequent eventual incapacitation.

The necessity to maintain autonomy in relation to criminal justice is even stronger in the case of social dangerousness. This category, lacking any psychiatric significance, is nevertheless used to justify the restraint of a mentally ill offender, declared incapable, within the confines of penal justice. In the absence of 'secure' civil psychiatric institutions a pronouncement of social dangerousness can seem attractive to the court, not only in the case of serious offences, but also in cases of widespread and repeated disorderly behaviour, of that petty criminality which disturbs the public peace and often contributes more to the general anxiety about crime than do individual serious offences.

Here too forensic psychiatrists tend to carve out for themselves an area of specific intervention. Once the evaluation of dangerousness has been disconnected from any diagnosis of illness two strategies become available. The first seeks to redefine dangerousness as the probability of recidivism in relation to the presence of a certain number and type of 'risk factors' (Ferracuti 1986: for a similar position discussed with respect to the United States see Mauri 1988). Forensic psychiatrists become epidemiologists who deploy statistical analyses to assess the probability of the defendant committing further offences starting from the interaction of factors seen as productive of risk, presumably for a personality already judged to be 'ill' – even if, as has already been seen in the United States, this is a procedure extendible to all 'criminals'. What characterises this position is the implicit assumption of the existence of a measurable tendency to criminality.

The second strategy, conversely, anchors the prognosis of dangerousness in the case by case evaluation of the viability of treatment of the individual in the context of his or her social surroundings. The tasks of forensic psychiatry become more complex as the prognosis of dangerousness is simply the starting point for bringing the psychiatric disturbance into relation with the material life situation of the individual. Forensic psychiatry then takes on the task of suggesting and identifying the types of treatment which, in its opinion, can reduce the probability of recidivism.

The principal client of forensic psychiatry remains the criminal justice system and it is really in relation to the increasing and contradictory demands of the courts that psychiatrists are driven to defend their disciplinary and professional autonomy. Innovations in psychiatry are deployed to give substance and authenticity to this autonomy. The demands of the criminal justice system are, on the other hand, presented by the forensic psychiatrists as relevant in contrast to the dominant therapeutic vocation of clinical psychiatry, which is often reproached for not being willing to take on the problems of social control. As we can see, one way for forensic psychiatrists to respond to the innovations both in clinical psychiatry and in the field of penal reform is a reinterpretation of one's expertise such as to extend and reinforce the sphere of competence of the profession.

On the level of practice, this process of reinterpretation takes the form of an often conscious effort to mediate among different exigencies. An indication of this is the proliferation, in psychiatric reports requested by judges, of diagnoses of 'partial mental defect'. Such diagnoses are, to say the least, dubious from the psychiatric viewpoint but they go some way to meet conflicting demands. The first of these is the argument from much contemporary psychiatry to the effect that diagnoses of total mental incapacity are anti-therapeutic. Second is the demand by both psychiatry and liberal public opinion concerned with 'due process', for the maximum limitation – if not the elimination altogether – of pronouncements of social dangerousness, with consequent limitations on the power of the courts to commit to penal psychiatric hospitals. Third is, of course, the argument of social defence itself for incapacitation as a justification for continued incarceration of offenders.

In this way diagnosis is arrived at[14] increasingly through socio-political rather than medical considerations: a further indication of a forensic psychiatry sensitive to psychiatric innovations, and yet which must however provide the court with a diagnosis. This in turn contributes to the proliferation of descriptions of 'borderline' situations, accounted for through the combination of diverse symptoms ('transitory dissociative psychotic episodes connected to aggravated neuroses', 'grave anomalies of the personality due to a fragile neurotic disposition', etc.).

Thus, the contemporary practice of forensic psychiatrists is characterised by an attention to the diversity and richness of the personal, social and environmental factors interacting in the lives of those they examine, and such diversity and richness is easily to be found in written reports. Yet, such practice does not always escape the traditional vicious circle of forensic psychiatry and the criminological knowledge derived from it, in which crime is assumed to be a symptom of psychic disorder and psychic disorder a factor in the outbreak of criminality. The breaking of biological determinism frequently takes the form of a tautology, or of a sociological determinism which in the final analysis coheres with the new demands of the courts and with the fundamental inspirations of penal reform. This is confirmed by the decisive importance which the criminal act acquires in the prognosis of social dangerousness. Such prognoses are infrequent and disconnected from a diagnosis of mental illness as such – there are schizophrenics declared incapable but not dangerous. Dangerousness is often contextualised – if appropriate care measures are available then the defendant will not be dangerous. But it remains anchored to the gravity of the offence: as if the expert could only oscillate between preoccupations with social defence on the one hand and rejection of referral to penal psychiatric hospitals on the other.

In fact the mandate of the forensic psychiatrist remains contradictory notwithstanding, and perhaps indeed by virtue of, attempts at its reinterpretation, and this becomes evident in professional practice. Diagnosis, the only real product of this practice, works as a straitjacket for the new, therapy-oriented psychiatric consciousness. The exclusion of a therapeutic role gives the appearance of objectivity to psychiatric reports which is difficult to reconcile with the inevitable complexity of the routes whereby they are arrived at.

RISKY CHOICES

On the juridical level the question of criminal responsibility (and liability to punishment) is linked to the retributive idea of punishment as moral censure presupposing 'free will'. It has then been argued (see Pulitanò 1988) that the concept of responsibility is in crisis today not only because of the crisis of the scientific nature of the assumptions on which such responsibility depends – in the Italian system, the presence or absence of 'infirmity of mind' – but also because modern penology is distancing itself from the 'retributive idea'. Criminal responsibility nevertheless remains as a fundamental cornerstone of criminal law inasmuch as it postulates a free will which is 'the standard of a consociality in which each individual can be recognised as a subject and recognise other subjects with equal dignity' (Pulitanò 1988, p. 128).

The crisis, which permeates both aspects of criminal responsibility, the normative as much as the empirical, is revealed in the decisions of individual judges. The ways in which institutional uncertainty is individually acted out are indicators of the judges' culture and are expressions of different options not only of criminal justice policies but also of social policies. Also, these different ways are related to how each judge perceives one's role, to changes in professional standards and to the presence or possibility of contacts with other institutions and agencies. Today many judges are well aware that their decisions regarding criminal responsibility are not 'mandatory', from the standpoint either of empirical investigation or doctrinal certainty; but involve explicit choices based on their political attitudes towards criminal justice and social policies (see Canosa *et al.* 1987; Gandus 1988).

Judicial decisions are then 'oriented to consequences', i.e., they take into account the possible effects of the different decisions themselves. This orientation is not only implicit, nor is it always denied by the judges. In many cases it is a conscious choice, in all it is present as an often difficult dilemma. It is a dilemma in which different exigencies conflict: exigencies relating to due process, among which are also those concerning the judicial role and its ethics (judicial autonomy, primacy of the law); conflict with substantive 'justice' exigencies; preoccupations with social defence, which often involve the desire to be legitimated by public opinion; conflict with the requirements of an equitable outcome in all those cases where referral to a penal psychiatric hospital is felt to be an exaggerated penalty.

One has, on the other hand, the impression that it is really the present situation regarding penal psychiatric hospitals, both from the practical and theoretical standpoints which makes the choices of the court particularly problematic. The courts complain of the absence of places which are both 'secure' and at the same time acceptable from a therapeutic point of view. It is this that imposes on them the search, on a case by case basis, for compromise solutions, which take account not only of the gravity of the offence, but also of the knowledge and evaluation of the antecedents of the accused, the availability of other agencies and institutions of care and the predicted reaction of public opinion.

To sum up therefore, from the standpoint of judicial practice the crisis of relations with psychiatry makes itself evident above all where the decisions concerning criminal responsibility and dangerousness are translated into choice of sanction. It can be hypothesised[15] that it is the latter which, in fact, determines the first: or that it is often the preference for a particular sanction in a specific case which influences the judge in the choice of an expert who will arrive at the desired conclusions as regards responsibility and dangerousness.[16] This probably always happened to a greater or lesser extent. What appears to have changed is that today this choice is seen as both deliberate and problematic. In this context the juridical debate on criminal responsibility is both uninfluential and a consequence, rather than a premise, of the problems concerning choices of sanction.

The recourse to the expert becomes more frequent, and no longer mainly in cases where a psychiatric syndrome is evident. But what is not clear is whether the courts require the expert to give explanations or to give rationalisations.

THE DILEMMA OF THE COURT: PUNISH OR CURE?

The courts do not have a great awareness of the law on psychiatric reform.[17] There is a reluctance to come to terms, at least explicitly (practice, especially that of the lower court judges, is another question), with a situation rendered unstable and fluctuating by changes in the psychiatric and penal fields, connoted by the interaction between a tendency to individualise punishment and the delegitimation (the disappearance in psychiatric care for the non-criminal mentally ill) of institutional and custodial solutions for mental illness. Such reluctance on the part of the courts is in part due to the distrust in the viability and effectiveness of the new community based psychiatry, but it is also, and perhaps most importantly, associated with a defence of one's own institutional competences. Notwithstanding the substantivist orientation of the last twenty years and the corresponding diffusion of intense political and social engagement on the part of judges, legitimation is still demanded in terms of a restrictive definition of one's role. Rather, it is this restrictive definition which is invoked by the judiciary to explain and justify its protagonism. (I refer to the polemics around the delegation to the judiciary of the handling of the political question of terrorism; and at the present time, the even stronger polemics concerning the so-called interventionism of judges towards politicians accused of corruption and fraud). This restrictive definition is emphasised all the more when judges have to intervene in the management of a social disturbance which is diffuse, fragmented, and capable of provoking public alarm.

This restricted definition is defensive and often contradictory, as is evident from an analysis of responses to a questionnaire distributed to judges of the Milan court as part of the research project mentioned above.[18] The unease of the minority of judges who responded is revealed in the contradictory nature of their responses. Thus much is expected from psychiatric reports notwithstanding the declared distrust in the scientific objectivity of the categories on which the experts are called to pass judgement; there is a distrust in the possibility of scientific ascertainments of social dangerousness, while the expert is nevertheless expected to determine its extent and declare him- or herself convinced of a connection between dangerousness and at least some forms of mental illness; and opinions clearly critical of the penal psychiatric hospital are accompanied by a simultaneous desire to maintain it as a locus of 'therapy'.

At a more detailed level, among the minority of judges who completed the questionnaires two tendencies, at times intersecting though more often distinct, are noticeable. Each of them is expressed by more or less the same number of respondents. An account of these two tendencies can usefully start from the responses to the questions concerning attitudes to the proposed introduction, in the Italian penal procedure system, of a 'criminological' expertise. This is, in a certain sense, a watershed question: those who responded negatively underline the risks inherent in a criminal law oriented to the offender rather than to the offence, and identify themselves with a legal culture emphasising the separateness of the discourses and competences of criminal law from those of the social sciences. Those judges who, by contrast, saw criminological expertise as a necessary tool to come to terms with the increased complexity of the situations confronted by the courts, seemed to have in mind, even if only on the practical level, a new and more extensive concept of integrated penal science.[19]

Even the first tendency however, at least as it is expressed in the questionnaire responses, adhered to a notion of integrated penal science: but it is the traditional one in which the social science utilised is exclusively psychiatry and in its purely diagnostic role. Psychiatry is nevertheless not conceived of as only useful to the judge in the area of 'due process' (the ascertainment – albeit in conventional terms – of the capacity or otherwise of the defendant's fitness to plead) but with respect to the classification of 'types of perpetrators' as is confirmed in the advocacy of its utilisation for the ascertainment of social dangerousness.

The two tendencies cannot therefore be outlined as the one restrictive and oriented to 'due process' and the other substantivist and expansive. Rather, beyond the issues already alluded to, the adherents of the second tendency seemed to express a much greater unease than the first with regard to their own proper competence. The call for criminological expertise seems to indicate a desire for the acquisition of more and increasingly complex information on the context in which the offence takes place in addition to information on its alleged perpetrator. On the other hand psychiatric expertise is already currently utilised as an instrument for the contextualisation of the crime and its perpetrator. Those who reject criminological expertise seem largely to trust, or hope, that such contextualisation will lend support to a clear psychiatric diagnosis, freeing in some way judges from the burden of arriving by themselves at a decision which, although it must be based on the offence, takes account of the offender and the context. In designating the offender as the object of a psychiatric diagnosis, the judge would remain formally the judge of the act.

Judges who are in favour of the introduction of criminological expertise thus exhibit a higher level of confidence (or hope) that the social sciences may be able to handle the issues concerning the offender and his or her environment. These judges are, on the one hand, well aware of the difficulties of contemporary psychiatry in this regard, but on the other, entertain the hope that other social sciences can contribute to the formation of a 'scientific' diagnosis (judges in the survey were almost unanimous in requiring precise expert clinical judgements) which nonetheless maintains the focus on the two issues of incapacity for intentional action and social dangerousness.

On these two crucial points there were significant oscillations and contradictions within the same individual questionnaire response. For example: one judge maintained both that incapacity is an 'inherent characteristic' of serious mental illness and at the same time that its clinical and scientific foundations are highly debatable. Another respondent regarded the penal psychiatric hospital as a necessary institution for the functioning of criminal justice and yet that there is no need for places of physical confinement for the mentally ill. Others agreed that social dangerousness does not have 'a secure scientific foundation' in psychiatry (and that the penal psychiatric hospital should be abolished) but yet demanded from the psychiatrist 'circumstantial evidence on the dangerousness of the (mentally ill) subject'. These contradictions indicate a generalised uncertainty concerning both the impact of the increasingly problematic character of forensic psychiatry and the consequent difficulty of maintaining the conventional boundaries between the proper tasks of the judge and the expert. The question of the penal psychiatric hospital is symptomatic and the responses on this point give the impression of both a pragmatic attitude and a desire for secure albeit 'dignified' solutions to the problem of the mentally disabled offender.

Nearly all maintained that the most important reason for retaining the legal category of partial mental defect was that of avoiding incarceration in penal psychiatric hospitals. This attitude underlines the lack of viability of the present system of penal psychiatric hospitals and the widespread avoidance of recourse to them by the courts. But in reality the demand is not so much for the abolition of these hospitals as for their transformation into purely therapeutic institutions. There is here, besides an implicit diffidence towards the law on psychiatric reform, the desire that judicial and therapeutic competences be completely separated. The possibility and desirability of such separation is, however, linked to the availability of custodial solutions, even if for 'therapeutic reasons'.

These attitudes are of course to a considerable extent a product of each judge's culture. But it is important to ascertain how far such attitudes are also a product of contacts with community psychiatric services. We know[20] that such contacts are rare, haphazard, and not part of normal procedures. There are many judges who would like the forensic psychiatric expert to provide, in addition to diagnostic classification, recommendations as to possible therapeutic solutions thereby implying the possibility of treatment in the community. For these judges, then, the presence or absence of such possibilities seems to be important in terms of the decision regarding sanctions. This in its turn implies a more extensive conception of the tasks of the expert than simply that of diagnosis, however fundamental the latter. The expert comes to be seen in the role of mediator between criminal justice and clinical psychiatry or, rather, between the relative chances of criminalisation and therapy. Is there here an implicit admission that judges are participants in the management of social disorder alongside other agencies? – that the separation between judicial and therapeutic competences refers rather to the institutions than to the object of these institutions? The fact that the capacity for intervention of non-criminal justice agencies becomes a factor in court decisions seems to be a move in this direction.

THE DILEMMAS OF COMMUNITY PSYCHIATRY: TO PUNISH IS TO TREAT?

The various psychiatric services instituted by law 180 operate with very different models of intervention in different parts of Italy. This is a product of differences in organisational resources, in the political and cultural environment in which the services operate, in the training and professional culture of the practitioners, and naturally – always important in Italy – the geographic area in which they operate (see the CENSIS research).

I will describe, briefly, three examples of intervention and the relations between the psychiatric and health services and the criminal justice system involved. These three differ among themselves, but they are all in one way or another 'advanced' with respect to the general situation in Italy as regards the implementation of the reform legislation. Milan, Trieste and Perugia, in fact, went through a long period of experimentation and innovation prior to the legislation itself. In Trieste and Perugia the services 'function'; that is to say they have sufficient resources, trained and motivated workers, and are open or available on a 24-hour basis. In Milan (see Micheli, Carabelli 1986), the situation is not as rosy, but is nevertheless better than in other areas of Italy.

It should be added that in Trieste there is an elevated unity of purpose and orientation between individual services, even if they are differentiated in terms of client groups and resources. In Perugia the three community mental health centres adopt distinct models of intervention and in Milan the differentiation is even more accentuated both in relation to the breadth of users, the diversity of problems they present, and the orientation of the practitioners. Here, however, my focus is on the forms of relationship between these services and the criminal justice system, in terms of how they operate with regard to that 'grey area' of problems at the boundaries of the two systems, and how they manage the respective responsibilities and competences.

It has already been said that the professional culture of psychiatry is currently characterised by an orientation to therapy. Nevertheless the meaning of therapy and the models of treatment and care are quite diverse. It seems possible to identify two principal models which are sometimes separated and sometimes combined in the same service. The first model develops the therapeutic orientation in a restrictive way, purging it of any allusions to social control, by basing itself on mainly 'medical' resources (pharmaceutical, psychotropic drugs of various types) and producing, as a consequence, a restrictive definition of its competence. Obviously the type of clients served are, by definition, those who present problems compatible with the medical models deployed, that is, problems of a 'purely' psychiatric nature which can be theorised in terms analogous to the 'symptoms' of other illnesses. The standard of psychiatry becomes in principle that of general medicine. Supply determines demand, in the sense that the latter, in order to receive a response, must be formulated in terms compatible with the supply itself. There is, thus, a double process of selection: on the part of the services and on the part of the client.

In the second model psychiatry is seen as a frontier discipline in which therapy takes on board all the problems which the old asylum contained and concealed. The object of psychiatry remains 'impure', and includes problems of various origins and nature, and requires a pluralism and flexibility of techniques and approaches. Tasks of social control are consciously assumed and developed as part of the management of problems ('disturbances') whose complexity and multi-dimensionality is fully recognised.[21]

Services based on this model tend not to select cases on the basis of psychiatric symptoms abstracted from context but to embrace a wide variety of both cases and methods of intervention. Thus pharmaceutical and psychotropic drugs of various types are accompanied – as an integral part of the treatment[22] – by various forms of welfare and social work, liaison with other welfare agencies, development of work experiences for patients.

Both the conditions of existence of the two models and the concrete forms they take are determined by the resources effectively available together with the cultural and political context in which they operate.

The extent to which tasks of social control are consciously assumed is determined by the models of service delivery derived from the inter-connection between particular therapeutic cultures and the organisational, political and economic relations which influence how agencies define their responsibilities. In the custodial model, these tasks, justified by the concept of dangerousness ('to oneself and to others') of the mentally ill, implied the absence of rights for the 'incompetent' – in other words the exclusion of any preoccupation with reciprocity or treatment by consent and a regime in which the responsibility of the professional was concerned exclusively with custody and surveillance and negated any responsibility on the part of the patient. Today patients have become clients, citizens for whom the right to treatment is recognised. This right changes the tasks and the respon-sibilities of the psychiatric professional, implying an obligation on his or her part to respect the will of the client in providing treatment.

It is here that psychiatry reveals its distinctness from the dominant models of general medicine.[23] The psychiatrically disturbed are often resistant to treatment because they are themselves unaware of the disturbance from which they suffer, a factor that is often compounded by the fact that such disturbance is only one aspect of a problematic situation in which family conflicts, lone-liness, poverty and perhaps the abuse of alcohol or other drugs combine. Here psychiatric disturbance implies a situation in which the requirements of social control appear problematic to the professional. The need for treatment is wide ranging and can go unrecognised by the potential client and is articulated rather by the family, by neighbours or by the agencies of public order themselves.

The professional finds him- or herself facing a dilemma. If in principle the client's right to treatment appears as a professional obligation, so does the requirement to respect the client's 'free will' (for an analysis of the contradictions inherent in this status of the client and of the implications for the professional standards of the worker, see Dresser 1984). The dilemma is additionally complicated by the simultaneous demands arising from those surrounding the client and from the agencies of public order. The problem then appears not so much that of whether or not to include the task of getting the client to agree to treatment as inherent in the role of the therapist, but rather as how far to respond to the externally imposed requirements of social control and social defence; issues which have little to do directly with the problems of the client.

There are different ways of understanding and confronting this dilemma. The two models of service emphasised above refer precisely to two radically different solutions, which imply the adoption of different therapeutic paradigms with their respective conceptions of the tasks of professionals and of the object of psychiatric intervention. Naturally, in the work of social service agencies, these two models do not present themselves in a pure form and have to be understood rather as the outcome of interaction between therapeutic cultures and organisational, political and economic constraints than as coherently followed choices.

In the Milanese case (for a more detailed analysis see Gallio 1988 and Micheli, Carabelli 1986) the progressive impoverishment of resources and the rigidification of organisational constraints helped to constrain the Psychiatric and Social Welfare Centres (*Centri Psico-Sociali*) towards a distribution of resources characteristic of the first model. In Milan interventions do not go beyond the agency itself, they are directed to the individual client at the time and for the duration which the client requires and are offered within a traditionally oriented ambulatorial programme, and they imply typically 'psychiatric' orientations (pharmaceutical, psychotherapeutic). The external interventions are delegated *in toto* to the social worker, in a division of labour in which the latter assumes the status of 'critical conscience of the service' (Gallio 1988). But the psychiatric tasks themselves come to be divided between the service and the hospital based diagnostic and care teams with emergency cases being delegated to the latter and handled through the institution of Compulsory Medical Treatment[24] with responsibility being thus removed from the social workers. The fragmentation and specialisation of professional competences intensifies selectivity of the clientele: clients are only accepted whose problems are compatible with the modes of treatment on offer.

As Gallio puts it

> . . . the consequences of this model . . . are to be seen in terms of a series of refusals when the demands for control predominate. Refusal to intervene when it is not the client in person who applies to the service, but others such as neighbours who make the request. . . . Refusal additionally to take responsibility for clients labelled as socially marginal (drugs addicts, alcoholics, those from public hostels etc.) when psychiatric symptoms are not held to be prevalent. Refusal to intervene when the problem is seen as one of 'behaviour' and conveyed as such by those requesting intervention.
>
> (1988 p. 250)

This series of 'refusals' is, on the other hand, justified by the services in terms of the necessity for psychiatric services to distinguish themselves from other agencies of social intervention and from those of public order. The result is that the refusal becomes the paradigm for a new psychiatry whose object is purified of historical contamination by social marginality (Gallio 1988). The *de facto* isolation of the Psychiatric and Social Welfare Centres becomes an isolation *de jure*, vindicated by reference to exigencies and demands perceived as extraneous to its proper competences and responsibilities.

It is hardly surprising, therefore, that the contacts with the agencies of public order and the criminal justice system as a whole are rare, sporadic and casual. The scarcity of clients with criminal problems which we ascertained through the reading of a sample of clinical records at the three Psychiatric and Social Welfare Centres in Milan is attributable to the way in which the services tend to reject or ignore this type of client rather than to an absence of problems of this type in the area under consideration. The service takes in only those who enter voluntarily and tends to follow them only to the threshold of other agencies, including criminal justice. Patients who run into trouble with the law vanish, the professionals ignore what happens to them unless, rarely, someone (the trial judge, the lawyer, the investigating judge) requests information, or the client reappears spontaneously after a period in prison, or even in a penal psychiatric hospital.

It is not, however, this small quota of clients with criminal problems who form the nub of the relationship (or rather non-relationship) between the psychiatric services and the criminal justice system. The character of the relationship is underlined by potential clients who do not appear because they lack the right prerequisites to be taken into care. These are the people who circulate between the public hostels, the police cells and the court, or who suddenly appear in situations of crisis, conflicts in the family or with neighbours or who become involved in public disturbances resulting in intervention by the police, or who are arrested frequently for brief periods, but who can also at some point end up being sent to penal psychiatric hospitals.

Interpretations of one's own competence and concrete choices have an impact precisely on this 'grey' area, on its extension and destiny. Isolation of the agencies from one another and tendencies to a restrictive definition of proper competences mutually reinforce one another, aided by a lack of information and a climate of mutual suspicion. If the courts often lament the unavailability or the lack of structures of welfare and care, and blame these for their decisions to send people to prison or penal psychiatric hospital, welfare professionals point to the impenetrable structures of the criminal justice system, often attributing to these the disappearance of their clients. In the middle are other institutional actors such as the police on whom falls the task of sorting out and handling these types of problems. Above all, the reciprocal isolation of the various agencies can only contribute to the exacerbation of moral panics and demands for the exclusion of those seen as threats to social order.

In Trieste there has developed over the years a different model (see Mauri 1983). The mental health services operate with an orientation towards the outside world, developing a diversified array of interventions in which welfare, promotion of work and leisure oriented activities, and therapy in the strict sense are indissolubly intertwined. There is very little selection of the demand, such as to embrace crisis and chronicity, psychiatric illness and social marginality. The services at Trieste form a network of interventions on a variety of levels – diagnosis and treatment, centres for drug dependants, group accommodation, work co-operatives, etc. – functioning over the full twenty-four hour period, integrating multiple skills and developing organic relations with the other institutions and agencies. That has allowed the formation of a group of practitioners who work permanently in the prison (Novello 1987), and the construction of a dialogue with the courts which tends to involve the services in decisions concerning the destiny of the client who runs into trouble with the law. The new Italian penitentiary and penal regulations are taken by the psychiatric services workers as a terrain in which to experiment with criminal justice practitioners' interventions which do not sacrifice the right to treatment to social defence concerns. Such a situation however pre-supposes that the psychiatric practitioners are available, as well as being in a position to take in charge difficult and often highly risky situations and to share responsibility with the criminal justice system. Such cases imply particular obligations both towards the individuals taken in charge as well as towards the demands for protection by the collectivity. Such a strategy of intervention implies reciprocity. It is not a question of substituting for other agencies, accepting matters delegated from them but rather working to develop collaboration, mobilising the professional skills and fostering the commitment of all the actors involved.

The terrain is in fact slippery, all the more so where the legal context is uncertain and the boundaries of the proper competences unstable and controversial. The recent experience in Perugia is a good illustration of the problems and the risks involved in such a situation.

In Perugia, a city where the experience of new psychiatry preceded the reform of 1978 and took the form of Mental Health Centres very active in the community and supported by local consensus among citizens who had been directly involved in the process of de-institutionalisation, one of the psychiatrists in charge of a Centre was recently convicted of neglect of a mentally disabled person. This conviction is curious and at the same time emblematic because the 'disabled' in question was not himself a client of the Mental Health Centre but the son of a client. The story was, briefly, as follows. There was a family, parents and two sons, riddled with conflicts and tension, a situation of which the neighbours were well aware. The mother was undergoing treatment at the local Mental Health Centre whose practitioners were making frequent home visits. In the course of these visits the tense situation in the household was noticed by the practitioners so that the psychiatrist responsible drew the attention of the police to the situation albeit on an informal level through personal contacts. During a period of admission of the mother to hospital, one of the sons killed the father in the course of an argument. The arrest, trial and conviction of the psychiatrist (the case is still subject to appeal) was based on the attribution to him of responsibility for not having intervened in the situation to prevent the homicide. The issue here was basically that of the attribution to the mental health agency of tasks which went well beyond the 'normal' assumptions of the requirements of control in situations of risk. The agency, in the person of the psychiatrist responsible, was invested with the global responsibility for whatever occurred in the situation in which it was intervening: including tasks of surveillance, prevention, policing – not only of the client but of the entire situation in the household. It was a total delegation to the Mental Health Centre as a substitute for other agencies and responsibilities.

This is precisely the risk run by agencies like those mental health services which for reasons of culture or history are not locked into the specificity of the clinic, and so do not segregate psychiatry from the 'murky' aspects of welfare, control and hence of marginality, poverty and deviance. The risk of substitution is then experienced as the attempt to unload on the service everything which 'causes problems' in the community. This can lead, on the part of the service itself, to a defensive rigidification and to a restrictive redefinition of its proper competences.[25]

The episode described above is probably an exceptional case, but it is a good illustration of the presence of conflicts between different agencies and institutions. A 'weak' psychiatric service can contribute to a hypertrophy of the intervention of the agencies of public order, which in their turn contribute to reinforcing this weak identity; but the unloading of responsibility to the 'strong' services – a potential consequence of this strength itself – risks either the 'psychiatrisation' of the community, or a defensive closure, the self-isolation of the service within rigid and reduced boundaries.

It is within this network of reciprocal fear and defensiveness, that attempts to provide and share proper professional standards in the context of a fluid and uncertain situation and open or implicit conflicts which often play themselves out in individual cases, lead to the redefinition – on the level of practice even more than on that of theory – of the relationship between psychiatry and criminal justice.

RISKS AND DANGERS

The personal and institutional propensity to run risks varies inversely with the level of social perception and definition of danger. I define the latter as the subjective experience of situations which threaten one's own security, individual and collective. What such situations are depends on what is meant by the term 'security', the latter, in its turn, being correlated with sex, social class, geography and the structure of work and family relations. What is considered dangerous by a woman is different to what would be considered dangerous by a man of equal economic and educational level. The vulnerability to certain types of threat is not homogeneously distributed, as many studies of victimisation demonstrate (see for a discussion, Hanmer and Saunders 1984; Lea and Young 1984).

Nevertheless the experience of victimisation and the awareness of threat and insecurity are not directly correlated. An important piece of research conducted in a multi-ethnic area, characterised by widespread poverty and a high crime rate, in a large American city, (Merry 1981) reveals how fear, and hence the definition of what constitutes danger, is strongly influenced by factors such as the level of familiarity with the area, the degree of contact with neighbours, the existence and the practicability of relations between families and between ethnic groups, the existence and the frequency of use of social services, etc.

More generally, the perverse correlation between collective perceptions of danger, and resulting defensive strategies such as the desertion of certain areas, locking oneself up at home, not going out in the evening, and increases in the actual risk of victimisation indicates the importance of policies which confront issues of criminality and violence – not directly, through 'defensive' strategies legitimated by fear of crime – but rather through a process of empowerment involving the activation of various institutional competences and responsibilities, with the aim of promoting and supporting the participation and organised intervention of community groups. Such policies, rather than justifying themselves by reference to the existence of 'dangers', seek to define concretely and in practical terms what are the risks and who should be, and is, able to deal with them.

Risks and assumptions of responsibility are connected. The judge who decides to discharge the multiple killer declared incapable of intentional action but not socially dangerous, takes on a responsibility which carries notable professional risks. The same is true for the forensic psychiatrist and the social services professional. The closure of each within the confines of a rigidly and reductively interpreted professional competence diminishes the range of risks which each takes responsibility for, but also, through the processes of off-loading and withdrawal, multiplies the number of threatening situations, and increases the appeal of purely defensive strategies thereby diminishing the general social tolerance of 'danger'.

The personal and institutional availability to assume risks is higher in situations where there is collaboration and reciprocity. The risks are in these cases shared and are thereby reduced through the process of joint involvement and sharing of responsibility.

DIFFERENT SOLUTIONS, NEW PROBLEMS

In drawing together the thread of what has been argued up till now I will try to highlight some of the consequences relating to the different ways of handling the institutional uncertainties produced by the changing relations between psychiatry and criminal justice. A way of clearly separating the psychiatric and judicial spheres of competence, which seems to be favoured by many judges, is the separation of the trial process into two distinct stages. In proceedings of this type two levels of criminal liability (see Pulitanò 1988) would be distinguished. In the first phase, only the attributability of the criminal act to the suspect would be ascertained. In the second phase, when sentence is decided, the psychiatric opinion on the mental state of the convicted would intervene. Supporters of this solution argue that it would avert problems indicated by both psychiatrists and judges. There would no longer be the need for a psychiatric diagnosis of the capacity or otherwise of the accused to plead, but only an evaluation of possible mental disability, and a verdict of incapacitation, with its anti-therapeutic consequences, would be avoided. The judges would remain sole judges of the facts in the first phase, and only in the second, at the point of sentencing, would they have to take account of the personal history of the accused. That would avoid a situation in which the orientation to consequences determines the entire court proceedings.

The two-stage trial would institutionalise and regulate, what now occurs as a practical compromise between judges and forensic psychiatrists and which typically in the Italian courts results in the verdict of 'partial mental defect'.

This proposal is certainly in line with the logic of recent legislation relating to punishment, with the introduction of differentiated and flexible punishments. And in effect the two-staged process would obviously concern all defendants, not only those suspected of mental disability. The evaluation of possible mental disability would become only one of the aspects to be taken account of in deciding punishment. The second phase of the trial would deliberate upon what was the best punishment for a certain defendant and would thus utilise not only psychiatric, but also sociological and criminological knowledge. It is in this type of proceeding that the criminological expertise we discussed before would find its applicability: investigations of the personality and the history of the accused would be conducted and demanded for all defendants with the aim of finding for each one the appropriate sentence.

As far as the mentally disabled are concerned, the proposal is compatible, in principle, with the aim of abolishing penal psychiatric hospitals and entrusting the mentally disabled offender to local community based psychiatric services. However it seems more plausible to understand it as a proposal that, by legitimating punishment as treatment which can be differentiated in accordance with the 'needs' of individual offenders, is compatible with a wide spectrum of solutions, from confinement to a protected and secure place, to treatment while at liberty, all justifiable on the basis of the individual requirements of the case. On the other hand, as long as the dominant form of punishment remains incarceration, the consequences of a proposal of this type, for actual policy, would only be nominal: existing institutions would be re-defined as 'treatment' oriented. This, of course, already happens. It is on the basis of an already existing 'rehabilitative' and 'treatment-oriented' prison regime that some argue for the uselessness of penal psychiatric hospitals, and propose to convert them into exclusively therapeutic institutions (see Daga 1985). Whether they should become a particular type of prison, or, since the prison also 'cures', a particular type of 'cure', is not very clear.

The 'new' psychiatric expertise previously described risks moving in this direction. The route via the reconstruction of the history of the accused and the context of his action, the anchoring of the prognosis of dangerousness in the prospective outcome of treatment and welfare can be translated, as already noted, into a variety of sociological determinism even more susceptible to discretionality than traditional biological determinism. If history, context and situation are to be understood as explaining the crime, as 'causes' of the act itself, there can be a reduction of the accused to his/her 'needs' which is in no way different from the reduction to his/her illness. A similar consideration of 'needs' which can be extended not only to the mentally disabled, but to all criminal offenders (in complete conformity to the idea of punishment as treatment) can only lead to the legitimation of differentiated unequal punishments according to the type of offender. This, besides emptying the institution of criminal liability in any sense, and thus also of its implications as regards due process and the rule of law, would reinforce criminal justice policies oriented to the requirements of social defence and supported by a concept of social dangerousness far more extensive than that based on traditional positivistic presuppositions.

The relation between criminal law and social science would thus give way to a new 'integrated penal science', with criminology, sociology and psychology added to psychiatry in the robes of ancillary disciplines to law at whose disposition they would furnish scientific justifications. Meanwhile the penal system and social services would form an integrated network of institutions in which the diffusion of control, rather than being dependent on the distribution of resources, would be the principal task delegated from the penal system itself which would occupy a central place in the network.

But there are different ways of taking account of the history and concrete situation of the offender. As far as the mentally disabled are concerned, a psychiatric report is possible which attempts a reconstruction of the social and institutional context within which to decipher the meaning of the criminal action without reducing the latter to an effect of the former. History and context may be retraced in order to restore the concrete and complex dynamics which constitute the terrain – rather than the causes – of actions, rather than of behaviour. History, context and situation may be engaged with and analysed as constraints which, rather than annulling intention and 'will', constitute elements of it. An expertise which adopts such an approach presupposes a different way of interpreting 'needs' and points to different forms of relations between criminal justice and welfare (see Dell'Acqua, Mezzina 1988).

In translating concretely the right of all citizens to treatment, the psychiatric services can utilise the spaces opened up by the new prison regulations. The latter oscillate between a resocialisation paradigm and a rehabilitative and treatment one, and actually tend towards the latter, in conformity with the criminal justice policies within which they operate. They are, however, sufficiently contradictory to permit practices which experiment with a resocialisation approach. Among these, the establishment of stable links between the prison and the outside world, the construction of routes from the prison to the outside world and the shifting of emphasis from treatment to resocialisation, can mobilise the flexibility of punishment from a preoccupation with forms of differentiation oriented to the aims of discipline and social defence into an instrument for the attainment of a complex equality (Walzer 1983).

The problem, in fact, is how to take charge of 'needs' without ignoring rights, something which cannot be done if a deterministic reading of needs is adopted, either of a biological or sociological type. Policies based on such an understanding result, on the individual level, in an incapacitating form of welfare and, on the collective level, in criminal justice policies oriented to social defence and the predominance of disciplinary models.

Conversely, the space exists, as demonstrated by the concrete actions of institutional and social actors, for a relation between criminal law and social science, between criminal justice and social and welfare services –

and also other institutions and groups such as local authorities, schools, trades unions, voluntary groups – which does not reduce the second to supports or sources of legitimation for the first. This is possible on different levels. The respect for individual rights implies the recognition and attribution of responsibility to the actor regarding the consequences of her actions. This in turn implies that the action itself is contextualised in terms of the constraints arising from the interrelation of personal with institutional and social events. The deconstruction of this interrelation is, in turn, an operation in which analysis and concrete intervention of the involved institutions must proceed together and must involve the active participation of the actor. These are the tasks of the social sciences and of the social services and welfare system.

Such tasks do not give rise to a new integrated penal science, because they do not provide explanations or justifications: criminal law works with an autonomous logic and discourse which elaborates in its own terms that which arises out of other forms of knowledge. Such tasks, on the other hand, would not create a disciplinary continuum with the prison at its centre, since they would imply involvement in specific processes of de-institutionalisation.

7 From oppression to victimisation
The debate on the Merlin law

In this and the next chapter I examine the events surrounding two pieces of legislation which are lucid illustrations of the political, cultural and legal aspects of questions concerning the regulation of sexuality, and in particular of the sexuality of women. It is unnecessary to say that the regulation of sexuality is a crucial aspect of the social control of women (on this see Pitch 1988, Introduction). There are, however, also other issues which come to light with the struggles around these two laws: the relation between protection and autonomy, the symbolic use of criminal law, the construction and the attribution and assumption of the status of victim.

It is no accident that the significance and consequences of these issues differ in the two series of events under consideration. In the first, the debate, during the 1950s, on the Merlin law on the regulation of prostitution, the objects of legislation – prostitutes – were not empowered to speak as such and neither did there exist a women's movement which took on this struggle as its own, as happened in the second case during the 1970s, that of struggle for a law against sexual violence.

Many things changed from the first to the second situation. But the questions relating to sexuality and especially that of the social relations between the sexes and the place of women in a male society, seemed to set alight passions and feelings which, though they expressed themselves in different languages, re-emerged in the (male) political and cultural debates in the second period, preserved almost intact from the first. What, by contrast, underwent profound change is the way women themselves posed and discussed the issues even if many of the problems and some of the solutions remained the same.

INTRODUCTION

In the debate on the Merlin Law – abolishing of the regulation of prostitution[1] – themes were presented which, in different terms, resurfaced during the 1970s: the relation between law, custom and morality, the prerogatives and the limits of state intervention, the unstable equilibrium between civil rights and the requirements of social defence. While, during the 1970s, these themes seem to have been imposed on Parliament by the force of public debate, during the 1950s the trajectory was rather the reverse. But in both cases the course of struggles around issues of custom and morality is particularly tortuous when women are both the objects and the subjects of these struggles.

The divisions, on the Merlin law as on later struggles around divorce, abortion and sexual violence, cut across the traditional political alignments. The left – the Italian Communist Party (PCI) and the Socialist Party (PSI) – took an abolitionist[2] stance as did, generally, the Christian Democrats (DC) and the Republican Party (PR). Against abolition were the Monarchists, the Neo-Fascist MSI, the Liberal Party (PLI) and the Party of Socialist Unity.

But the arguments of the various groupings cannot be interpreted on the basis of unified and coherent cultural models. On morality, sexuality, the family and women, ambivalent and often contradictory points of view mingle within similar positions towards the law. Furthermore, in the course of time arguments and terminology tended to change. The emphasis of the abolitionists, almost without distinction of political allegiance, became more moralistic, defensive and less preoccupied with 'high' political themes.

What was said at the time about prostitution and its regulation is more interesting for the interweaving of themes which it exhibited than the specific details of the debate. From this point of view it was an impoverished debate, and increasingly so as it progressed into the 1950s. Who were the prostitutes and why women turned to prostitution (less was said about why men sought prostitutes) was a theme which, predictably, was set forth in the parliamentary debate with little audacity and even less imagination. The abolitionists were paternalist, the voices of women being, for the most part, absent. The right was cynical and scientistic, though residual Lombrosian themes found an echo even among the abolitionist ranks.

I do not believe that it is a matter, in this as in other issues concerning women and sexuality, simply of the reductive and ambiguous effects of tactical alliances among different political formations. Alliances of this type are never purely tactical. There were serious and profound convergences between feminists and the militants of the crusade for social purity in the English abolitionist movement of the second half of the nineteenth century, in the same way as between radical feminists and the 'Moral Majority' in the campaigns against pornography in the United States.

In a situation such as the one under discussion where there is not a social movement, but rather a political alignment, the question poses itself in a different way. But it is similarly, if more extensively, connoted by sub-terranean convergences which cut across party lines and allude to a deep-rooted common culture. The ambivalences, the conceptual poverty, the silences, the apparently contradictory attitudes of the Left are traceable to a cultural background which is the same, in large measure, as that of the Catholics. This identity will gradually make itself heard more strongly as we move further from the 'high' moral climate of the immediate post-war period, and as politics gradually achieves its autonomy from personal and private contexts. One can also argue with good reason that the change in emphasis depends at least in part on changes in the social position of women during the ten years of the passage of the legislation: in 1948 still fresh from the experience of the anti-fascist resistance, projected outside the domestic sphere by the necessities of war, by the end of the 1950s succumbing, at least on the level of ideology and dominant culture, to the great return to the home.

ABOLISH REGULATION OR ABOLISH PROSTITUTION?

Angelina Merlin, a socialist senator, presented her draft bill 'Abolition of the regulation of prostitution, struggle against the exploitation of prosti-tution and for the protection of public health' to the presidency of the Senate on 6 August 1948. The complicated passage of this bill was con-cluded only after ten years, and a good two years after the parliamentary approval of the law on preventative treatment for venereal diseases. It was indeed quite a long period of time if one considers that the law finally voted did not differ from that presented in July 1949 by the Legislative Com-mission of the Senate, and that the latter already had, on paper, a large majority in Parliament.

The texts to be examined are therefore only three: the original project of Senator Merlin, the text redrafted by the Senate commission – definitively approved by the two houses of Parliament (as law no. 75 on 20 February 1958 – and the legislation (law no. 837) of 25 July 1956) on the prophylaxis of venereal diseases.

Lina Merlin's proposal was presented as an integrated project, con-fronting together issues relating both to the abrogation of the regime of tolerance and exploitation of prostitution, and to the 'protection of public health'. It was the second part that provoked the most heated discussions. It was easier to hide real opposition to the spirit of the entire project behind a veneer of objections relating to public health, with their secular, modern and scientific 'objectivity'. The public health aspects were in fact imme-diately separated out and referred to a separate committee, except that then, in the course of the debate of the new text presented by the Parliamentary

Commission in 1949 the opposition objected to its approval on the grounds that it lacked the public health aspects. This was then the first fundamental difference between the original Merlin project and the law of 1958 based on the text presented by the Senate Commission in 1949.

Let us begin with the original project of Senator Merlin. The pre-occupation with the abolition and prevention of any type of registration and recording – for whatever purpose, even the 'protection of health' of the women themselves – was fundamental, as was the related attempt to remove coercion from the issue of health visits and medical treatment. In the Merlin draft bill these dispositions are stated early on in article 2. The other fundamental objective is the struggle against the exploitation of prostitution. This was the concern of article 1 which prohibited the running of brothels, and article 3 which elaborated a compendium of all the possible forms in which exploitation was to be understood, besides the issues concerning the 'trade'. Procuring thus became a separate offence, subject to penal sanction even when it involves an adult woman, in full command of her faculties and consenting. This is a crucial point, to which I will presently return.

For the 'protection of public morals and human dignity', besides the abrogation of a series of measures contained in the law on public security, the Merlin text makes it a crime to 'invite into libertinage in a scandalous or molesting way' or pursue 'by any means persons in such a way as to cause their molestation'. It adds however that persons stopped in such a context, if they have with them regular identity documents cannot 'be detained by the police for further identification', neither, if without identity documents and therefore taken to the police station, can they then be forcibly obliged to undergo health checks. The successive articles of the bill from 7 to 10 are explicitly aimed at preventing any type of recording in police files.

The Merlin text then continues with provisions concerning the protection of 'public health'. Such protection is not to be obtained through the violation of 'human dignity'. There are two principal aspects: the abolition of the identification of a special population at risk and the attempt to avoid any form of compulsory treatment. Connected to these aspects is the removal of any competence on the part of the police as regards health questions, a theme which is further confirmed in article 18, which abolishes the so-called morals police and provides for the creation of a corps of women police 'devoted principally to the prevention of juvenile delinquency and prostitution'. Article 19 provides for the creation of Educational Institutes for ex-prostitutes managed by the local authorities. Access to these, it is emphasised, can only be on a voluntary basis and the institutions must provide 'for the instruction of the said women with the aim of a professional qualification'. With a similar peremptoriness the text concludes that brothels must be closed within forty-eight hours of the coming into force of the law, that the contracts of the women working in these houses must be considered extinct, and that these women themselves, at the closure of the brothels, must be interviewed by the police 'in the presence of women from welfare agencies who will give all possible assistance and protection.' In addition, 'in the shortest possible time the male medical personnel practising in venereal disease clinics during the hours of frequentation of women must be substituted by female medical personnel'.

The report with which Lina Merlin presented her draft bill revealed a civic passion which would gradually dissolve and dilute itself into a generalised moralism in the debates on succeeding drafts of the bill.

There are two focal points of this report. Firstly, at the end of the fascist period, the arbitrary and extra-legal activities of the police, the constant threat to privacy and personal liberty which the system of regulated prostitution symbolised appeared to the socialist Merlin as intolerable. Secondly, a theme which paradoxically would, at least explicitly, drop out of the debate, the equality of the sexes and the demand for dignity and conscience by women and their right to that equal liberty and possibility of social participation which the Constitution granted. There are by contrast few references, in this first draft, to sexuality, the family and to prostitution itself – themes which will later come to assume a central relevance.

Lina Merlin began by recalling three articles of the new Italian Constitution of 1948: the equality of the sexes, the prohibition of compulsory medical treatment injurious to human dignity, the inadmissibility of commercial enterprises which cause damage to liberty and human dignity. To these articles are closely linked, she argued, three objectives of her draft bill. The elimination firstly, of the private 'procuring of adults', secondly, of the regime regulating prostitution, a regime iniquitous in itself, as well as being a symbol and pretext for abuse of all women, and thirdly of an unjust – and inefficient – system of protection of public health based on the registration of prostitutes, health visits and obligatory treatment for venereal diseases. Prostitution, said Merlin, cannot be considered a crime: first of all because the autonomy of the person is a fundamental good and the State must not interfere in the private and personal sphere of the individual, but also because, by punishing it as such, either the principle of equality of the sexes would be violated or 'Italy would be reduced to a penitentiary'. Neither, according to Merlin, is it right to punish 'the attitude of enticement' a matter which is ambiguous and susceptible to arbitrary action and abuses.

It is these themes, abuse, arbitrariness, policing, which recur obsessively throughout the report. Cases are cited of women stopped by the police, coercively visited, confined under suspicion of syphilis on the basis of mere suspicion, or of anonymous reports, of blackmail by the 'moral police'. There is a denunciation of the climate of oppression and discrimination and control to which all women are thereby subjected. The double standard of morality is stigmatised and mocked, men are accused of irresponsibility and hypocrisy. These, in fact, said Merlin, are the real goals of regulation: 'for men in general: to procure for themselves security and comfort in vice, enforcing the silence of any and every woman with the threat of police investigation, reaffirming, despite public declarations and constitutional principles, male privileges and sexual inequality'.[3]

Indeed, added Merlin, could it not perhaps be said that the legitimation of the brothel through the pretext of controlling health is what has been devised in order to keep women in slavery after the Declaration of the Rights of Man? And as far as public health is concerned, the system of regulation not only does not protect it, but in fact threatens it. Women ought to refuse, as citizens, says Merlin, to pay taxes for the maintenance of health arrangements which threaten them directly, both from the standpoint of personal liberty, and as regards health itself. The control of prostitution, in fact, frees the clients from any responsibility towards their own health and contributes to the spread of venereal disease among 'innocent' women and children. On the contrary, the preventative treatment of venereal diseases has to be guided by the principle according to which law 'in order to be law and not the legalisation of arbitrary actions' must be equal for all and represent the most certain protection of the citizen against 'excessive power of individuals and the abuse of authority'. Venereal disease therefore must be treated in the same way as any other contagious disease, and the 'search for the sources of infection' must be explicitly excluded, as it is based on the unacceptable premise that 'suspicion (of infection) is a wrong which has to be expiated through submission to ill treatment'. The sick must retain the right and the duty to cure themselves, where they so desire, with the doctor chosen by themselves, by means of free out-patient treatment.

There is here an unsolved problem: how to reconcile individual rights with defence against contagion? How, in other words, to avoid the abuse of obligatory medical treatment and at the same time affirm the social duty of 'not injuring oneself and others'? Merlin proposed the punishment of those who, by refusing treatment, deliberately constitute themselves as a danger. However, even in this case, any form of coercion and segregation is excluded and responsibility on the matter is entrusted to 'medical authority'. Proper prophylactic measures must take the form of an obligation to certify oneself prior to marriage and of providing serological proof on all occasions where a certificate of health was required (students, soldiers on national service, public employees, workers, etc.).

Thus Merlin concluded her concise and stern presentation: 'Today all Italian women, who so heroically fought against tyranny, demand, in accordance with the letter of the Constitution, the removal from the legal code of the Motherland of Law, of an intolerable blemish, demand that the full right of inviolability of the person and the protection of the law will be extended to all women, and demand the suppression of a shame that offends the national honour, human dignity and civic conscience' (p. 19).

Quite different is the tone and direction of the draft bill produced by the Senate Commission and presented to Parliament on 29 July 1949 and which, after various tribulations, passed into law in 1958. The section concerning the prophylaxis of venereal diseases was removed and transferred to other legislative proposals. The protection of civil liberties and equality between the sexes was given less weight. What emerged, instead, were moralistic overtones, and charitable and welfare aspirations, together with preoccupations with discipline and repression. If the project of Merlin was entirely aimed at the abolition of the legal regulation of prostitution insofar as it was a system of discrimination, policing and oppression, the Senate Commission aimed at the abolition of legal regulation because, in the final analysis, it could not achieve the abolition of prostitution as such, but this is what it would have liked.[4]

If the emphasis of the original project fell on the safeguarding of liberty and drew its strength from the Constitution, the new project underlined rather the effects of 'corruption', 'vice' and criminality which regulation produced. Article 3 of the Merlin draft was maintained but was relegated to article 7. The concept of exploitation was widened so as to include, among other things, 'whosoever, being the proprietor, or warden of a hotel, furnished apartments, lodging houses, bars, places of entertainment, or their annexes, or whatsoever other place of public access or use, tolerates the habitual presence of one or more persons who, within the same location, devote themselves to prostitution' and whosoever not only 'recruits' but 'assists' prostitution on the part of any person (it is to be noted that the 'women' of the Merlin proposal are here substituted with the substantive 'persons').

Strong emphasis is given to the part concerned with 're-education'. The provision and financing of institutes for the 'protection, welfare and re-education' of ex-prostitutes is no longer the responsibility of the local authorities but a task for the Ministry of the Interior, and nothing is said about the necessity of providing ex-prostitutes with some kind of 'professional qualification'. The institutes, including the private ones, are subjected to state surveillance and control. Even more explicit is Article 10 concerning young persons. The original project was concerned only with changing the arrangements of public security which discriminated between young people of 18 and under and those aged between 18 and 21. The latter, said Merlin, could not be received in protective institutions and 'were abandoned to their own devices or directly provided with a health service card'. The original project limited itself therefore to saying that all young women under 21 could be received into institutions. Here, by contrast, is article 10 of the Commission's proposal: 'Young people under 21 who habitually and completely draw their means of subsistence from prostitution shall be returned to their families, it having been ascertained that these are ready to receive them. If, however, they do not have relatives prepared to receive them and who offer secure guarantees of morality, they will be, by order of the president of the tribunal, entrusted to the charitable institutions indicated in the present article . . .' where it is clear that the approach is that of a disciplinary oriented welfare.

The vehemence of Merlin against the organs of the police is also rounded off at the edges: no longer is it a question of the abolition of the 'moral police', but of the constitution of a special corps of women who 'gradually and within permitted limits' will replace such police in the tasks of managing juvenile delinquency, and prostitution. . . . The report which accompanies this project, set forth by the Christian Democrat Boggiano Pico, underlined the changed basic objectives and the decisive shifting of the question on to a less irksome terrain: from that of a struggle for civil rights and equality to that of the provision of 'moral cleansing', where repressive and educative – welfare aims agreeably coexist.

There is no more shifting from this terrain. Apart from a few rare voices, Terracini (an unorthodox Communist leader) for example, the left and the Catholics found a convergence on this terrain which was more than simply tactical.

Here is, then, the report of the Commission. At the centre not the legal regulation of prostitution, but prostitution, defined as 'the most shameful scourge of human kind', a social sore resulting from deprivation, the culture which imposes on women virginity up till the point of marriage, the brute passions of men. But also the result of heredity, the hypersexual temperament and the depraved nature of certain women. Traditional moralism seeks legitimacy in the form of an 'objective' and 'scientific' language. It is the scientism of common sense, a superficial Lombrosianism which makes recourse to 'biology' in the manner of the provincial petty bourgeois intellectual (the doctor and the lawyer).

Thus, the 'causes' of prostitution are both individual and social. Probably they are rather more social, but it is found necessary to add that once these have acted to push women to prostitute themselves, it is women who, 'after the break-up of the constraints of chastity', are the driving force in enticing and corrupting men, no longer because of poverty but from the 'desire for lucre', or, let's admit it, because of their 'hypersexual and depraved' nature. Prostitution is to be condemned 'not only from the ethical stand-point' but also from the 'biological' one. Biology has already demonstrated that 'plurigamous' relations are irrational for the human species. The human instinct is distinct from the animal because whereas the latter is oriented by '*libido coeundi*', the former conforms to '*voluntas generandi*' (which indicates, among other things, that prostitution here does not mean only to exchange sex with money, but to have sexual relations with several people and for reasons other than procreation). State regulation is to be abolished not because it violates the civil rights of women but because it 'legitimates libertinism'. If it is desirable to affirm the 'ethical nature of the state' one cannot then allow it to facilitate and legalise 'vice'. The real remedy however (i.e., the remedy to prostitution), has to be sought elsewhere: through a more rigid discipline at school, sexual education, sport. As if to say: if we re-educate the instincts of (male) youth we will have no further need of prostitutes.

Some aspects of the law for the prophylaxis of venereal diseases (law 837, 25 July 1956) make a relevant comparison. In reality, notwithstanding its separation from the original Merlin proposals, the numerous conflicts and the long passage of the bill, this law did not differ so greatly from the orientations of the original Merlin project. To get oneself treatment is an obligation (there is a fine for those who refuse), but it is also a right: treatment is free and can be sought both at the appropriate clinics which the law provides for, and with a private doctor, or any other clinic or hospital. Hospitals are obliged to give treatment. Any doctor who becomes aware of the presence of venereal disease, in its contagious phase, must advise the Regional Medical Officer, safeguarding the identity of the patient. It is conversely a duty of the Regional Medical Officer, in particular situations, to ask doctors for the names of patients, and subject them to a health visit. If the supposedly ill person fails to present themselves, or is found to be contagious the Regional Medical Officer can arrange temporary isolation from the workplace and, in cases where the individual refuses, can impose obligatory admission in a hospital until the disappearance of the contagious phase. In all cases in which the presentation of a certificate of health is required, it must be ascertained that there has been a blood test for syphilis.

CIVIL LIBERTIES AND SOCIAL DEFENCE

The long duration of the parliamentary passage of the Merlin law cannot be explained by looking simply at what was going on in Parliament. In both the Chamber and the Senate the bill had, at least on paper, a large majority. Approved by the Senate in 1952, and by the Parliamentary Commission in the same year, presented again in the Senate at the beginning of the new parliamentary session (in August 1953) and delegated to the Senate Commission in deliberating session, it was newly approved in January 1955. From here it returned to the Commission of the house of deputies where it was discussed together with the law for the prophylaxis of venereal diseases. While the latter was approved, the Merlin bill was sent back for discussion in the Chamber's plenary session on the initiative of members in favour of regulation of prostitution. This discussion began with the speech by the Christian Democrat Tozzi Condivi in April 1956 and concluded only at the end of January 1958. Inertia, indifference, bureaucratic hindrances, but above all an extensive press campaign against the bill combined with the efficient work of the brothel owners in organising an effective lobby, all contributed to the delay.

In this matter, Parliament appeared as more 'advanced' than the country at large. Or rather, this is how the question was posed in the immediate post war period. The left explicitly maintained that Parliament (the state) must be a stimulus to innovation, democratisation and the cultural modernisation of the country. This was a much debated issue, which was solved in different ways.

For example, the maintenance (right up to 1981!) of crimes of 'honour' in the Italian penal code was conversely often justified (also by the left) by the difficulty of imposing 'modernisation' on certain local cultural areas by command from above. This type of attitude, in the case of the Merlin bill, came from the political right. It was argued that cultural attitudes had to change first, otherwise such legislation would bring about a series of disasters with regard to health, morals and public order – increases in venereal diseases to epidemic proportions, the diffusion of every conceivable type of vice and perversion such as homosexuality, 'onanism', adultery, sexual crimes, psychological illness deriving from 'inhibition of the instincts', and also, of course an increase in criminality and public indecency.

The arguments of the regulationists, were, predictably, as confused and contradictory as those of the supporters of the bill: but if the latter sought legitimation from high ideals – a mixture of civil rights, social justice and Catholic morality – the former made recourse to 'realism'. It was a realism that also fused together, with naturally opposite effects, 'science' and traditional culture. Science here appears in the form of medicine (the medical associations were in the front line against the law) and, in part, biology, which here was borrowed to reclothe common sense in authoritative garb. Thus while it was being demanded that the law await an 'evolution of customs', which would have to be brought about by a much invoked and very vaguely defined 'sexual education' in the schools, it was also being said however, that 'instincts' (of men) could not be restrained: we are after all in a Latin country, not in Sweden, and the (male) blood is hot! Prostitution is surely the 'lesser evil' – to homosexuality, onanism, etc. – besides being inevitable. And what was to be said, then, of the legitimate sexual rights of the poor, the old, the ugly, soldiers, sailors? Prostitution, thus, has important functions. But it must be controlled, for reasons of both health and public order. The state must not legislate upon morals: but it has the right, even the duty, to assume 'social defence'. The ethical state on the one hand, the pragmatic and interventionist state on the other.

In the face of these considerations, it is permissible to doubt whether the majority in Parliament were really more advanced than the country as a whole. What almost immediately occurred in Parliament – and in public debate generally – was an abolitionist battle continuously more marked by the defence and affirmation of traditional values (Catholic-conservative, respectable, petty bourgeois, and above all, misogynist). This struggle was part of a more general climate of 'moral' restoration in Italy during the 1950s (censorship of films, anti-pornography campaigns, defence of the 'sanctity of the family', the disapproval of sex outside marriage) to which a distinct secular morality failed to coherently counterpose itself. Thus the struggle against legal regulation and against prostitution – assumed by both the parties to the conflict as a symbol of a disordered sexuality, the source of 'depravation and corruption' – tended to become increasingly confused with one another.[5]

The cultural models proposed by the two sides were thus, from the standpoint of 'modernisation', both contradictory. Both propounded an image of the state which was, in different ways, heavily involved in the direction and management of the private life of citizens, the abolitionists, entrusting to it the task of ethical and moral leadership, while the regulationists (liberals included) entrusted to it the tasks of policing and paternalistic protection. The defence of civil liberties, the conception of the state as both supreme guarantor of the rights of the individual and promoter of social rights – a motive that inspired the original legal project, and which still shone through here and there in the parliamentary debate in the speeches of some of the left (Lina Merlin herself, Terracini, Riccardo Lombardi (a famous left-wing socialist)) – succumbed to the embrace of the Catholics. But it succumbed also by virtue of its weakness. The latter was related to a contradiction which, if it emerged clearly in the debate on Merlin, presented itself again in more mature forms in the political and legal culture of the 1970s and is a long way from being resolved. I refer to the double contradiction, typical of the welfare state, between individual rights and social rights, and between liberty and social defence.

Already on the issue of the recognition of pimping as a separate criminal offence, there emerged problems which were not easily resolved. The regulationists raised a curious objection, one which contrasted with the logic of their comprehensive attitudes towards prostitutes – who were frequently seen as biologically degenerate and physically retarded – and even more with their attitude towards the safeguarding of civil rights, which they constantly subordinated to the more highly prioritised requirements of 'protection' – of health, public order and social defence. Their objection was that the recognition of pimping as a crime was in conflict with the idea that adult women can choose entirely autonomously and freely to prostitute themselves. The original conception, that of Merlin, was preoccupied above all with finding instruments to strike a hard blow at exploitation and to achieve this end without hitting prostitution as such (rather like law 685 on drug dependency, in distinguishing dealers and consumers). There is no doubt however that the law, especially in its final formulation, lends itself to oppressive interpretations, impacting strongly on the everyday life of the prostitute (Teodori 1986), often taking the form of an implicit repressive protection. On the other hand, the interventions of many abolitionists, above all the Catholics, authorise a similar interpretation, in this case formulated in terms of the notion that women are weak and must be protected.

But it was around articles 5 and 7 of the bill (and then of the law) that the argument between abolitionists and regulationists concentrated, and it was within this discussion that the double contradiction mentioned above (that between civil and social rights, and that between liberty and social defence) revealed itself. These articles prohibit the imposition of compulsory health checks on persons stopped for infringements of the prostitution law itself, the detention by the police of persons stopped for enticement when they are in possession of identity cards, and of any form of registration or recording (be it even for health reasons) of women suspected of involvement in prostitution. The regulationists, and also the Department of Health (and therefore the government, favourable to the law), invoked the right and duty of the state to guarantee the 'supreme good' of public health, even at the cost of sacrificing 'the liberty of some'.

It is not only by invoking social dangerousness that the maintenance – or the re-establishment in other forms – of an exceptional regime for prostitutes was defended. Certainly, this was the main argument. Prostitutes were dangerous, inasmuch as a 'source of spreading of venereal disease' among themselves and to others and would therefore have to be subjected to a special health surveillance in the name of social defence. But there is another aspect which was raised even if in guarded tones. The closing of the brothels, it was argued, meant abandoning '4,000 unfortunates', for the most part ignorant, suffering not only from physical but also psychiatric illnesses, to the streets. There they would not only constitute a problem of public order and a danger to public health, but would themselves be deprived of any protection and care and without any guarantee of medical treatment.

The Merlin law – and above all the original project – frees, but does not protect either the public in general or prostitutes in particular. The contrived and mystifying form in which such arguments were formulated hardly deserves comment. The problem, however, in principle, is real enough and has practical implications. The final solutions adopted were two: the law on prophylaxis of venereal diseases and the already cited charitable institutes. The first, of which I have given some indication, introduces a form of obligatory treatment surrounded by such discrimination and caution as to give the impression that it was being introduced mainly in order to silence doctors and the political opposition. In this way a social dangerousness specific to prostitutes disappears, and this disappearance is legitimated by arguments about health care. However, such a strategy was possible precisely because prostitutes continue to be viewed as socially dangerous, not only according to the police and public security laws, but according to the notorious law of 27 December 1956 (law no. 1423) in which all those persons who come within the definition of 'persons dangerous to public security and morality' and in particular those who 'habitually pursue activities contrary to morality' are to be subjected to 'preventative measures' such as obligatory travel permits, special surveillance, confiscation of driving licence etc. (Pavarini 1975).

The second solution is based on a welfare-paternalism with explicitly disciplinary connotations. The 'redemption' of the prostitute is to come about through a process of re-education described in terms not dissimilar to those preached in connection with the prison – and often practised in the case of women's prisons (see Faccioli 1987). The task of 'moral elevation' through religious practice is to be accompanied by the 'hard discipline of daily labour'. The latter, in the absence of provisions aiming at the acquisition of any sort of professional qualification, can – and in reality must – only consist in traditional forms of female domestic labour. Hard labour as punishment with a purely disciplinary function.

Thus the problem is broken up into two, rather, three parts. Abolition of regulation in the name of obedience to constitutional principles and the safeguarding of the rights of individual liberty, welfarism conceived not as the response to social rights or needs recognised as legitimate, but as disciplinary re-education and social defence entrusted to the discretion of the police. The alternatives for prostitutes seem to lie between an oppressive welfare which has all the characteristics of enforced treatment (of the soul if not of the body) and being the object of public order measures largely left to the discretion of the police. Difference is reaffirmed as threat.

Because it cannot be clearly defined in terms of crime and punishment, it is consigned to a terrain where it is the simultaneous object of therapeutic measures (then of a 'moral' type, nowadays of an openly technical–medical type) and of police measures. It is a fate that befalls nowadays (at least at the level of intentions) all those areas from which the criminal justice system retreats, to which the alternative of abandonment and ghettoisation must be added.

FROM OPPRESSED TO VICTIMS

A struggle which was motivated by progressive secular values degenerated into moralistically repressive legislation. A fate shared by later struggles, those for divorce, abortion, and against sexual violence. However, in these later struggles there was an autonomous female voice which made itself heard and which, apart from the legislative results that were achieved, imposed new demands and opened up new contradictions. I will examine this voice in the next chapter. Here I want to conclude with some more general considerations of the conditions which make possible apparently heterogeneous alliances of the type illustrated in the conflicts around the Merlin law.

The first of these conditions seems to me a particular understanding of the theme of oppression. As I have noted in a previous chapter, the terminology of oppression is complex and any struggle oriented to legislation conducted in its name can only reduce and simplify it. The reduction works first of all in the identification of two separate chains of causes and effects. In the case of struggles concentrating on a single objective, however much it may be symbolic of a more general situation, the specific effects being fought against are accentuated and exaggerated. This has the effect of rigidifying and paralysing the struggle, but also of facilitating the entry into it of motives extraneous to the original inspiration, insofar as they appear to restore complexity to the objectives of the struggle. In the case of the campaign for the abolition of the legal regulation of prostitution, the condition of the prostitute is depicted in ever more extreme tones as the struggle advances – slave, pure commodity, victim of numerous forms of brutality, etc. Such a wretched condition, however, cannot be imputed simply to legal regulation, notwithstanding that this was the original focus of the struggle. Elements of it come to denote the condition of prostitution as such. If, on the other hand, the prostitute comes to symbolise the oppression of women in general the struggle, having portrayed that oppression in extreme terms by exemplifying it in the condition of the prostitute, has difficulty in moving from the particular to the general without at the same time opening itself to voices coming from other contexts which then contribute to isolating the specific effects of oppression symbolised by the prostitute by adding a new series of 'causes'.

Another contradiction has to do with a particular portrayal of the theme of victimisation. Its accentuation risks downplaying those processes of interaction crucial to the development of subjectivity and to separate and render reciprocally autonomous those who speak and act from those for whom the speaking and acting is done. The prostitute becomes the victim *par excellence*, the extreme limit of the oppression of all women, but for this very reason she has nothing to say, or at most, speaks only as testimony. We, who are not prostitutes, speak of her and for her, at first because it seems to us that her condition alludes to ours, but gradually as she takes on the role of victim, she becomes rather the object of our solicitations, of our benevolence, of our pity.

If these are some of the conditions which can be at the basis of heterogeneous alliances between women/feminists and 'moral majorities' of various types,[6] it is much easier to understand the convergences among traditional political forces of a diversity of inspirations: on the question of sexuality, of relations between men and women, the culture which, at bottom, unites them is not so different. It is a culture which, as we now know, speaks with the male voice.

If the first report accompanying the Merlin law was inspired by a coherently emancipatory attitude (full citizenship, equality between the sexes, work opportunities outside the home for women, denunciation of double standards of morality), the discourse which developed in the 1950s in the abolitionist ranks seems to have run over again through the steps of the English abolitionism of the 19th century, from feminism to the crusades for social purity. Women do not have to be liberated but defended. Prostitutes are fallen women, all the lower because women are sacred and elevated creatures, saints of the hearth and the guardians of the morality of the family. This was not only the discourse of the Catholics. The left did something more than come to an instrumental agreement. In large part it shared it and contributed to consolidating it. This type of emphasis can be found already even in the interventions of Lina Merlin herself in the Senate debates in 1949, in support of the project of the Commission. 'By nature,' said Merlin, 'every woman is a woman and every woman is a mother'. The distance between acting subject and 'object' for which one acts, accentuated by the absence of a movement, produced in the later years distortions in this sense. Merlin assumed the not quite secular status of 'saint', 'mother', and 'apostle' of prostitutes (see Merlin, Barberis 1955).[7]

8   From victimisation to autonomy

Women, feminism and the law on rape

Some aspects of the legislation on sexual violence in Italy have been discussed in chapter 4. There my concern was with the convergence of the struggle for legislation on sexual violence with other struggles in respect of what I termed a symbolic use of criminal law and, contemporaneously, the emergence of a particular mode of assuming and attributing 'responsibility'. It was by means of this latter, I argued, that actors were brought back into the picture: as abstractions, free of constraints, mere bearers of rights. But this story is more complex and here I shall examine its contradictory aspects, highlighting that richness which a translation into questions of criminal law risks obscuring, and with which in reality, as I have already hinted, it enters into tension. It is precisely this tension which is my interest here, both because it concerns the difficulty of reducing concrete individuals to simple (and 'equal') bearers of rights, and because at the same time it signals the presence of different and contradictory demands for the assumption of responsibility.

There is a specific character to the issue here – that concerning relations between the sexes – which distinguishes it from analogous events involving subjects whose demands for 'difference' stand in contrast with simultaneous demands for 'equality'. It is, however, worth asking whether such demands for the recognition of 'difference' would not be better understood by reference to this much more radical and irreducible 'difference' which underlies and cuts across all the others.

BY WAY OF A PROLOGUE

There is no woman who does not understand the fear of being raped, who has not been sexually molested (a smack on the bottom, the wandering hand), who has not been subject to sexual innuendo and insults, to obscene jokes. Many women, many more than one knows or suspects (American statistics certainly speak of a third of all women), have suffered serious sexual violence: many of these in their own homes, from fathers, husbands, brothers, boyfriends.

It is only recently that such things have been talked about. In common opinion, still, in legislation and even more in the administration of the law, in the court room and in the police station, sexual violence is seen as the product of a perverse sexuality, sick, abnormal. Violators are a category of males apart, different from other men. A condition for the existence of such sexual violence, for it to be recognised as such, is that the woman who suffers it must be eminently credible. But, to be credible she has not only to show that she did not want contact (better if she can show bruises, scratches, wounds, blood, etc.), but also to not be the type of woman who 'invites' violation. And this in its turn can mean many things. That you have to be 'respectable', or not sexually 'promiscuous' (it is difficult for a prostitute to be violated: is she not, already public property?), that you are supposed not to know the man who rapes you and even less to be on affectionate terms with him – real violence comes from perfect strangers, on the streets, while of course you are going to work, shopping, on your way home: never that you are just taking yourself for a walk, even less alone and at night! Such behaviour is already suspect. Don't even speak about being so stupid as to accept a lift, or even worse to ask for one. . . . To behave in a way which is not 'provocative' is extremely difficult when anything can constitute provocation, short skirts and long ones, tight trousers, net stockings, walking in a certain way, smiling in a certain way, looking a man in the face, etc., etc.

Here is the credible woman: she leaves the house alone only during the daytime and by well populated streets – better, however, if she is accompanied, and always for definite purposes; she is dressed in such a way as not to catch the eye; she keeps her eyes rigorously lowered and never smiles; she is either a virgin or happily married, either a housewife or has a respectable job (teacher, secretary, clerk): she does not drink nor make use of other drugs. She is credible, naturally, if the violence which she reports is inflicted by strangers, better if more than one, and if it has left visible marks on her body. Even this woman is not credible if she complains of having been violated by her husband, father, boyfriend, in her own home. We know today that the greater part of the violence is really of this type. From four-year-old girls to women of ninety, at home, in the workplace, in the street, by boyfriends, relatives, parents, husbands. But who knows it, and how do they know, and what does it mean to know?

Women who report, and above all those who report their own fathers, husbands, boyfriends, of having raped them, are few, but they are increasing. What does this mean? That they are few can be read as an indication of the fact that (a) these are things which happen very rarely; (b) that women know they will not be believed; (c) that women are frightened of reprisals, or even more simply, that they are economically (and emotionally) dependent on fathers, husbands, men they live with, employers, etc.; (d) that it is not easy for women themselves to recognise, name, perceive what happens in certain situations as sexual violence because the dominant culture does not recognise it as such, and also because the association between sex and violence is extremely strong, legitimated culturally, interconnected with the traditional subordinate position of women in the family and elsewhere.

That they are growing in number can be seen as an indication of the fact that (a) sexual violence is increasing; (b) that women know that they have an increasing probability of being believed; (c) that women have less fear of reprisals and/or they are less economically (and emotionally) dependent on their own fathers, husbands, men they live with; (d) that the emergence of a feminist culture has made it easier to recognise, name and perceive what happens in certain situations as sexual violence.

Sexual violence is not rare at all, it is frequent and common. Even when women have not said it, literature, history, the very history of the prohibitions against rape say it.1 Its effects show it: women's fear, the internalisation of attitudes and the clear adoption of types of behaviour (not going around alone, not speaking to strangers, not responding when pestered), which are implicitly subdued and defensive; or an a *priori* dependence (he is my husband, escort, employer). This is what makes for complicity (perhaps I provoked him?) a complicity made stronger by the presence of the relationship, perhaps of affection. But there is no doubt that what is seen as sexual violence, the perception of actions and events taken as constituting violence, have changed with the development of a feminist culture, and that this is, and was, a potent factor in increasing the credibility of women, in giving to women increased possibilities of recognising, perceiving, naming the violence and of feeling that they will be believed when they report it.

What I want to say is that not long ago the majority of us would not have defined, perceived, or recognised as rape what we now define, perceive and recognise as such. Does this mean perhaps that therefore sexual violence as a thing in itself does not exist, or does it mean that before we were not aware of it and today we are? In the first case nothing exists before being perceived and named; in the second case everything is already there, and it is a question of discovering it sooner or later. In both cases however, the precondition for perceiving and naming, as well as for discovering, is to be in a position to see in a new way and to name in a new way. Both cases therefore necessarily imply a shift in the distribution of power, some dislocation in the social fabric, such that a series of individuals become constituted as 'we', and that this 'we' can acquire a voice and be listened to.[2]

If this 'we' says that violence exists, and that it existed before 'we' had the possibility of perceiving it and naming it, and that gradually as our position changed and with it our angle of vision, we perceive or discover increasingly more situations to be violent, the question of whether or not that is 'true' is a political question, a question around which conflict takes place.

It is a conflict a great deal more complex than any other. It involves in fact all the levels of experience and human existence, starting from our own (us as women, that is) affectivity, identity, from the foundations of our relations with others (women and men). It involves less the dichotomous opposition of identifiable actors (men, women), than the intersection of a plurality of different cultures and ideologies produced by men and by women. It does not create a single politics; rather, as I will seek to show, it should present and impose a diversity of political articulations charac- terised by openness and flexibility.

VIOLENCE OR SEX?

The traditional scientific literature on sexual violence, predominantly medical, psychological, criminological, tends to move within the following two hypotheses: either the violator is a pervert, or he is someone who has normal sexual instincts but is unsuccessful – or has not succeeded in the particular situation concerned – in keeping them under control. It is characteristic of this literature to focus on the actor rather than on the act. This presupposes that only confessed violators or those sentenced by the courts are to be studied, with the distorting effects well noted already long ago in relation to the researches of Lombroso on imprisoned criminals.

This literature, however, sees sexual violence as connected, and linked to, sexuality: abnormal in one case, normal in the other (in the theory of 'abnormality' often the 'real' culprit is seen as the mother, overprotective or conversely cold and rejecting; in the theory of 'normality' account has to be taken of what the language of the Anglo-Saxon legal tradition calls 'victim precipitation', the provocation by the victim herself). In both cases such events are seen as relatively rare and exceptional occurrences which entertain only a very vague relationship with everyday sexuality.

Already sociological research of the early 1970s (see the famous study by Amir 1971) has demolished certain myths: that sexual violence only occurred between strangers; that only young, attractive and/or provocative women were its victims; that rapes tended to occur interracially (the American mythology of rape – the black man who rapes the white woman – has fuelled the long history of lynching, see Dowd Hall 1983).

It is however the research linked to the emergence of feminist move- ments which has revolutionised what we know and what we think of as sexual violence.[3] Rather than summarise what is by now an abundant literature I will dwell on a point which is today more controversial, which has to do less with the phenomenology of rape than with the interpretation of its nature and significance. There are two dominant versions, predominantly Anglo-Saxon, concerning sexual violence. According to the first, rape is a variety of the phenomenology of violence: that it, in this case, expresses itself in the form of sex is, in the final analysis, secondary. Sexuality and sexual violence belong to two different categories. Where sexuality is a matter of consensual participation, shared pleasure, rape is an abuse of power, a form of expression of feelings and sentiments of hostility, hate, fear. However difficult it is to distinguish rape from 'normal' heterosexual relations – difficult from the, so to say, empirical standpoint – on the theoretical-interpretative level this position affirms that where there is rape there is no sexuality and vice versa. It is not at the end of the day a factual question, instead it is in some ways a matter of principle: this interpretation accepts that there are or can be heterosexual relations not characterised by coercion, and on the contrary presupposes that coercion and sexuality are mutually exclusive.

There is sexuality when there is 'consent'; violence or the absence of 'consent' cancel sexuality.

The separation of sex and violence and the consigning of rape to the latter, permits struggles against coercive forms of heterosexual relations while 'saving' heterosexuality as such by separating it clearly from those forms. The existence of a 'good' sexuality is thereby confirmed. On the more specifically political level, this separation has often served the need to oppose conservative interpretations to which sexual violence is seen as the result of a sexually permissive culture, moral decay, the fragility of the traditional family, female sexual freedom. It has inspired and favoured many demands for legislative change. If the criminal law already embodies this distinction, imposing rigid boundaries between normal and violent sexuality, the assigning of rape to the category of crimes of violence has been seen as a fundamental step in the symbolic recognition of women as 'equal' – as persons, rather than as 'sex' or 'morals'.

It is indeed a distinction which speaks the language of equality of rights – of emancipation – rather than that of sexual difference. The cancellation of the distinctiveness of rape as a violence *sui generis* cancels both its gendered character – the fact that it is an action of men against women – and its sexual character – the fact that it is enacted by means of sexuality. Sexuality itself is not discussed: its concrete historical modes of expression, the contradictions and the ambiguities with which we live and experience it are put in parenthesis with the result that good sexuality is deferred to the realm of the pre-social 'state of nature' where it functions as a presupposition necessary for the affirmation not only of the distinction between sex and violence on the basis of an existing consent, but above all of the very possibility of such consent.

According to Vega (1988), this reading refers to a framing of the question in terms of one of the two dominant philosophical formulations concerning the nature of rights, that of Locke. Heterosexual relations are seen as in themselves unproblematic, as 'naturally' free of power. Here violence is seen as a threat of or use of force in violation of 'natural' rights. The corollary is the possibility of a consent which is unambivalent, freely arrived at and clearly separated from coercion.

The second interpretation, by contrast, consigns rape to the sphere of heterosexuality (see Dworkin 1982; McKinnon 1987), whereby the latter is interpreted as violent through and through: the distinction between sex and violence is a fiction, as in reality violence is sexually stimulating and a source of pleasure (for men), while 'normal' sexuality is commonly violent without being for that reason any the less sexual. Normal heterosexuality, according to this interpretation, is constructed around the male pleasure in violating, overwhelming and dominating women, pleasure which requires the complementary female pleasure in being taken, dominated, and annulled as a person. This interpretation is not contradicted by the fact that women may experience this sexuality as their own, that they may be stimulated or experience pleasure in being violated or dominated: on the contrary this only proves the success, the pervasiveness of male culture, which has imposed its own sexuality as sexuality *per se*. The male point of view has become ours as women and therefore we cannot invoke 'consent' as a point of distinction between what is sexuality and what is violence because it is precisely the consent itself which is the problem: it is never free, but always marked by domination.

If, in the first interpretation, female liberty is a given fact of nature, in this perspective it does not exist at all: such that it is not at all clear how standpoints different from the dominant (male) view can emerge, how such an interpretation itself could have been articulated.

Rape is here both gendered and sexual: yet a woman's lived experience of heterosexuality is never 'true' when it is the source of pleasure, being the result of the total victory of male supremacy, of the interiorisation of male sexuality as her own – while on the contrary it is a fundamental mode of domination, the main instrument in the annulment of female liberty, of the construction of sexual difference as female subordination and inferiority. Here the dominant sexuality, heterosexuality, is regarded not only as a generic instrument of domination but also as being the specific vehicle of a violence which inscribes itself in blood on the bodies of women, of which rape is one side and pornography the other.

Heterosexuality is never egalitarian, it is rather constructed around male pleasure in overcoming and annulling, and on (the fiction of) female pleasure in being overcome and annulled. In this view, the feminine naming of the pleasures of heterosexuality is the entirely colonised discourse of an unwilling accomplice.

Also here, therefore, any ambiguity disappears: domination and freedom are incompatible, they exclude each other. In the first interpretation, female freedom appears as a fact of nature, the character of which is no different from freedom 'in general'. The female subject loses its female characteristics and dissolves into the abstract subject of rights of the liberal philosophical tradition (and modern political discourse). In the second interpretation, whereby feminine and masculine are constructed as mutually exclusive categories, the feminine only appears as the site and result of oppression. How female freedom can emerge, where it can be situated and the preconditions for the existing state of affairs to be revealed as non-natural and oppressive, is not clear.

To each of these two points of view there corresponds a partially differing interpretation of the 'functions' of sexual violence. The first view tends to restrict itself to the effects of intimidation, threat, self-censure (the policeman in the head) which confers on sexual violence the function of an instrument of control and repression of female autonomy – in the sense of having access to the same freedom of action as the male (see Brownmiller 1975). The second traces the effects of sexual violence and dominant heterosexuality well into the construction of male and female identity, as functioning to create and construct women in addition to maintaining their subordination. In other words, the connection between 'women' and 'subordination' is rendered inseparable.

Two ways of understanding 'social control' are in play which are partially distinct, but again have in common the placing of female freedom and autonomy beyond control itself, in opposition to it: in the first case, control can only be prohibition, censure, punishment; in the second case it is constructive of a subordinate, dominated, identity – of an identity which can only be conceived as inauthentic.

Naturally I am simplifying and stating an extreme form of these two positions. The analysis of the Italian debate will make visible some of the reciprocal contaminations, at times the contradictory co-presence of these standpoints.

TWENTY YEARS OF STRUGGLE

In all jurisdictions rape is considered a crime. What varies however are the definitions of rape, the legal procedures for conviction, prescribed sentences, attitudes and behaviour of the police, courts, hospitals, etc. Such variations concern not just legal differences but also the professional subcultures involved. Notwithstanding these differences, the laws, legal procedures, attitudes and behaviour of criminal justice professionals have been seen by the women's movements as detrimental to the rights of the victim, indulgent with regard to the rapist, weak in the definition of rape, generally complicit in, indeed supportive of, a culture saturated with violence against women.

Struggles for reform have been aimed at widening the types of behaviour definable as rape (in the United States, Canada and England and Wales for example to allow the possibility, until recently inadmissible, of prosecution for rape in marriage) and strengthening the position of the victim in the trial process (again in the United States, Canada and England and Wales for example, through the modification or the curtailment of the requirement for the prosecution to produce evidence of another individual besides the rape victim herself and to demonstrate that the victim had offered resistance, and the exclusion from admissibility of the sexual history of the victim as evidence against her (see Caringella-MacDonald 1988)). In general, these efforts have been directed toward the 'normal-isation' of rape, or making the handling of rape by the criminal justice system as similar as possible to that of other offences – changes pursued however, as will be seen also in Italy, for different motives by politicians, jurists and sections of the women's movement.

If many legal statutes have acceded to the changes demanded, it does not seem however, on the level of the figures for arrests and convictions, that things have changed significantly. Even more disappointing seem to be the results in relation to changes in the position of the victim. Even though excluded by legal statute, the requirements of corroborating evidence, of proof of resistance, of the admissibility of the sexual history of the victim are in practice alive and well (see Bienen 1983; Marsh, Geist, Caplan 1982; Snider 1985).

Undeniably however there have been real changes in common attitudes to rape (as shown by, among other things, the strong increase in the level of reporting), however much these changes meet with contradictions and resist-ance.[4] In many countries, campaigns for the reform of law and administrative procedures have been accompanied by other actions and political struggles. Telephone hot lines, Rape Crisis Centres, refuges for battered women, aware-ness training for police, hospital doctors, voluntary services in hospitals, etc.. Many of these initiatives and services, starting out as voluntary organisations of militants, have obtained official recognition and finance, and have taken on a professional character, becoming social service agencies in their own right. This has resulted in changes in the logic and practice of their functioning –

rigidification of rules, adoption of a therapeutic orientation, increased selectivity in acceptance (see Morgan 1981; Stark, Flitcraft, Frazier 1979) – which has exposed them to criticism by those who see them as new instruments for the institutional control of women.[5]

SEXUALITY AND MORAL CRUSADES

As already mentioned in relation to prostitution, the questions raised by sexuality constitute an arena for the playing out of interconnected conflicts concerning fundamental aspects of our lives: interpersonal, social and economic relations, and fears and expectations connected with them. This gives rise to what we might call 'grey' conflicts, struggles characterised by the intermingling of contradictory themes whose objectives can, in the medium term, be placed within differing and at times opposed, world views, and which then react on those same world views changing them in one direction or another and contributing to the creation of a 'hybrid' common sense in which aspects of each establish an unstable coexistence.

The debate on the sexual permissiveness of the 1960s and 1970s is illuminating from this point of view. Sexual permissiveness is denounced and opposed on various levels: by conservative pro-family forces and New Right movements as well as by some feminists on the ground that sexual permissiveness entailed the mere liberation of male sexuality and is the source of new forms of enslavement of women permeated by a consumer ethic.

One has the feeling (see Snitow, Stansell, Thompson 1983) that in the space of twenty years we have passed from the celebration of a liberated sexuality as an element of creativity, joy, of a truly revolutionary change, to a discourse which sees in sexuality only the negative: violence (against women and children), emotional disorder, and death (from AIDS). What certainly has happened is that there has been a new silencing, scarcely had they begun to speak, of the voice of women. The discovery or perception, by women, of the violence of the dominant sexuality, of this sexuality as not their own but imposed, has had neither resources nor time to stimulate research on sexuality, let alone for the development of new forms of sexuality.[6] Rather it has been merged with instances of prohibition and censure, or put on the defensive by attacks on contraception and abortion and by the medico-technological offensive in the area of reproduction (Stanworth 1987).

There are however other reasons, perhaps more important, for the female silence on sexuality, or rather for a discourse which develops only as a response to 'external' events and in terms and conditions imposed by others. Some of these emerge in the debate on sexual violence in Italy to which I now turn.

LEGISLATING ON WOMEN'S BODIES

Fifteen years have passed since a section of the women's movement drew up a bill for the reform of the law on sexual violence, launched by a campaign and petition to Parliament which gathered three hundred thousand signatures.[7] Today (January 1993) a new law on the issue, by now supported across the political spectrum, has still not been approved. The process is in danger of going on even longer than that of the law on the deregulation of prostitution, as if to confirm that issues relating to sexuality, while in the first instance concerning women, in reality put into question the relations between the sexes and the constitutive part they play in all other relationships. The mobilising impact of such issues goes far beyond the predictable political alignments to activate and throw into confusion a multitude of passions, fears and traditional equilibria.

But neither is there a compact female/feminist line up. Right from the beginning, this bill divided the women's movement, and gave rise to debates, polemics, analyses and taking of positions which over time have developed to create a rich, shifting, fluctuating scenario, in which rigid and inflexible standpoints are not easily traced.

These fifteen years can roughly be divided into three phases. The first started with the popular struggles resulting in the drafting of a bill signed by the *Movimento di Liberazione delle Donne* (Women's Liberation Movement), the *Unione Donne Italiane* (Italian Union of Women), the *Movimento Femminista Romano di via Pompeo Magno* (Roman Feminist Movement), and by *Coordinamento Donne FLM* (a women's co-ordinating group within the Metalworkers trade union), and concluded with the presentation to Parliament in January 1983 of a bill drawn up by a parliamentary commission and based both on the proposal arising from the popular initiative and those presented between 1977 and 1979 by all political parties.[8]

Over this period the debate among women centred around two main questions and two secondary issues which were to assume major relevance in subsequent periods. In reality these questions were conglomerations of problems rather than single issues, as will become increasingly clear. The first issue concerned the legitimacy of (women's) legislating on matters regarding (the bodies of) other women. It raised both the legitimacy of the principle of delegation or, as it has been called more recently, representation – in this case moreover self-assumed – and the possibility and legitimacy of the direct utilisation of the law as an instrument without the political mediations made use of during the campaign for the legalisation of abortion. Was it legitimate that women should legislate for, on behalf of, and concerning the bodies of other women, when up until then there had been a refusal to translate women's demands into politically negotiable objectives, as this implied the inevitable reduction of the ambivalence, the complexity, of their own analyses, their own desires and of their own battles (see Pitch 1983a)? Also, up until then, feminists had rejected the practice of delegation and representation among themselves.

Two elements merge into this critique of the promoters of the bill. The first is the anti-institutionalism of the women's movement. An institutionalism different from that of the 1968 movement: I called it elsewhere the practice of ambivalence, since it was characterised by a conscious practice of oscillation between acting within and outside the institutions (see chapter 3). The second was the critique of traditional forms of politics for which delegation and representation are fundamental.

On the other hand connected to this critique were the second cluster of problems, introduced through the debate on the nature of sexual violence. The popular initiative for legislation promoted the idea of rape as a crime of violence against the person, negating thereby both its gendered and its sexual nature. This provoked much dissent[9] which however shared neither the same terminology nor had the same outcome as the analogous debates in Anglo-Saxon feminism.

What was in fact challenged was the reductionism rather than the falsity of the interpretation of rape as violence. The discontinuity necessitated by the criminal law between legal and illegal, between violence and sexuality was what was criticised above all else: legal formulations were accused of the closure of an analysis before it had been completed; where the promoters of the new law defended its formulation as provoking consciousness raising, the dissenters accused it precisely of the opposite, of impeding the development of an autonomous analysis of sexuality from a feminine perspective. This critique did not start from a position which consigned heterosexuality to the catalogue of violence but rather from the perceived need to preserve the ambiguity of lived experiences, an ambiguity neither to be negated *a priori* nor to be interpreted as the product of male colonisation.

Several different issues are involved here. The rejection of the interpretation of rape as mere violence combines with the rejection of the law as an instrument seen as particularly reductive and over simplifying. The apparent universality of legal norms (rape is a crime of violence against the person) is interpreted as annulling the specifically gendered and sexual nature of the struggle and its aim: precisely what the promoters indicated as one of the main aims of their proposed law – or, the solemn symbolic recognition of the principle that women are 'persons' (and not 'morals').[10] The dissent appeared thus to be connoted by anti-reductionism: towards unidimensional interpretations of sexuality, towards the mechanism of the criminal law, and towards political campaigns which rejected such ambivalence. It was sustained also in opposition to tendencies which seemed to join feminist demands to campaigns for 'normalisation' and rationalisation led by 'secular and liberal' political forces who, sensitive to egalitarian and 'modernising' needs to eliminate from the penal code particular anachronistic laws and forms of legal protection,[11] worked for a definition of rape which would make it as similar as possible to all other 'normal' crimes.

There were in addition, throughout this period, critiques more internal to the proposals for the new law. Often advanced by feminist lawyers, involved in struggles concerning due process, against the use of imprisonment and for the reduction in the use of criminal law, they contested both the effectiveness of the criminal law as an instrument with regard to rape and what seemed to be departures from due process in the proposed new law (the weakening of the defence of the accused, the provisions for group rape, summary trial).

There were however two questions in particular regarding the formulation of the proposed law itself which gave rise to major conflict. The first concerned *procedibilità d'ufficio*. (Mandatory prosecution once a serious offence is reported – not necessarily by the victim). This the promoters justified by reference to two sets of arguments which, in actual fact, were in conflict with each other. Firstly in order to defend the woman from blackmail and relieve her from the *risks* of reporting the rape, secondly as a solemn confirmation of the gravity of the crime of rape by treating it as a crime to which society as a whole must respond (the first motive being based on the necessity of protection, and hence confirming the specificity of the crime as against women, the second based on the necessity of a symbolic recognition of equality).[12] These were criticised by the dissenters also from various standpoints.[13]

The position which by contrast argues *querela di parte* (proceedings initiated by the victim) as generally expressive of the liberty of women, was in fact still not widespread despite increasing prominence. At this time, this position had not yet been clearly articulated from a theoretical point of view so as to distinguish it from the apparently similar demand for respect for women's self-determination. This latter demand, during this period, was conflated with a concern to allow the woman who had been victimised the freedom not to put herself through a humiliating trial and at the same time to avoid the constraints of political trials. There is here a re-elaboration of the idea of female weakness: it must neither be forced, nor defended by institutional measures. Rather such weakness must be considered as a resource and a stimulus: a resource, where it expresses rejection and distance with respect to the existing system, and alludes to a complex experience not comprehensible within the confines of traditional politics, especially when the latter is played out within the criminal justice system. A stimulus in that it calls for a showing of female solidarity such as to render whatever choice is made, a free choice. Oppression and its effects are not negated, but there is a refusal to use traditional remedies against it, that two-faced politics of equality – assimilation and of protection as withdrawal of autonomy which the demand for mandatory prosecution seemed to embody.

The second question, relating to the provisions contained in the proposed law which foresaw the possibility of civil actions by associations and movements oriented to the liberation of women has two interconnected aspects. On one hand there is dissent again from the standpoint of the freedom of choice of the individual woman who demands legal action: the rejection, in a word, of a political trial with its potential prevarication from the standpoint of the victim. On the other hand, what is criticised is precisely the implicit objective of the proposal (see Pitch 1983a): the demand for political recognition by the official institutions, especially since it came to depend on characteristics extraneous to the movement, such as having a statute and being a formally organised association.

These were the issues around which the debate concentrated within the women's movement in the early years. Elsewhere (Pitch 1983a, 1985) I have analysed more thoroughly the arguments of the proposers for the new law and the political and social background within which the campaign developed and involved large numbers of women, a large proportion of whom, up to that point, had remained outside the feminist movement. There is no doubt that it was this side of the movement, favourable to the presentation of the bill as the principal arm of struggle against sexual violence, which had the highest public profile, was more influential in official politics, more capable of mobilisation. From the attendance of militants at rape trials, through the writing of the draft proposal for legislation and the organisation of a petition, the sponsoring of large demonstrations, the sustaining of a network of relations with members of the parliamentary commissions: the sponsoring committee for the popular initiative for a new law on rape certainly did not introduce into Italian feminism any 'new forms of politics' – on the contrary it was frequently accused of accommodating and unthinkingly reinforcing the traditional rules of the game – but at least it gave a framework to the desires of many women for political action in the pursuit of a 'simple' objective, already translated into politically negotiable terms, and of which the achievement could be easily controlled.

If this was an aspect of the success of the campaign, it is also linked to the fact that the objective was a modification of the criminal law, and here I refer to the analysis already developed in chapter 3, concerning the simplicity of the objective, its strong symbolic valence, its putting in parenthesis and simultaneous evocation of the cluster of problems of which it had become the symbol.

THE FEAR OF MEN

The second phase coincides with the presentation and the passage through Parliament, in October 1984, of the text, recently revised, of the draft legal reform bill, modified by the parliamentary legal commission and delayed by the fall of the previous government, and with its subsequent passage to the Senate in 1985.

This draft, like that from which it was derived, took up many of the proposals of the popular initiative for legal reform. Besides the replacement of Title XII of the Italian Criminal Code (crimes against the person), it envisaged mandatory prosecution in all cases, the unification into a single subject of rape and indecent assault, summary trials in open court, the specific crime of group rape, initiation of civil actions (for compensation) by associations and movements. It maintained however, in contrast to the original popular initiative for legal reform, the matter of presumed rape in the case of sexual acts involving minors under 14 or between 14 and 16 when the offender was the parent or guardian, unless it was a case of consensual sexual acts between minors with an age difference of not more than four years.

But the law which was finally approved by the Chamber (with the Communist Party, Independent Left, and Proletarian Democracy voting against) differed from the draft proposal of the parliamentary commission on several fundamental issues. It retained in fact *querela di parte* (proceedings initiated by the victim) in the case of rape between spouses or cohabitees, introducing such a double standard into Italian law for the first time. It re-introduced the presumption of violence in cases of sexual relations between minors even when the participants are of the same age, and in the case of sexual relations between handicapped and mentally ill; it denied the right of civil action by movements and associations.

The passing of this law also re-ignited the debate among women. In this debate some of the elements of the previous phase virtually disappeared. First of all, the distance between feminism and 'institutions', between inside and outside, was much less felt. The creation of an inter-parliamentary women's group as a protagonist in struggles in the Chamber and in the Senate on these issues, tended to function as a link. The movement could no more be conceived or function as 'actor', but as a diffuse culture, a diversity of initiatives: politics, public institutions, the social arena in general became a terrain of experimentation. One influential feminist theory argued that it was precisely the involvement of women in 'social intercourse' that led to the experience of their own irreducible difference which, if it emerged as 'unease in social intercourse' was in reality a resource if it was utilised to construct vertical relations between women, feminine lineages indispensable to a project of 'symbolic inscription of sexual difference' (see Libreria delle donne di Milano 1983). Though this type of theoretical development proceeded from the experience of a particular group – in this case the Libreria delle donne di Milano – it nevertheless found a wide diffusion because it valorised rather than stigmatised women's participation in 'social intercourse'. Even if misunderstood by many as a stimulus to the search for social affirmation, social success, it however transformed into something positive the diffuse demand by women to exist and to count, to start from the results of emancipation rather than to continue to bemoan the effects of oppression.

In this way, 'getting your hands dirty through involvement with the legal system' was no longer a point of conflict (at least, not a fundamental one) even if the law involved was a criminal one. Rather, while attitudes to the criminal justice system lost those connotations of mistrust and rejection adopted along with other things from the radical tradition of the 1960s and 1970s, there began a reflection on the nature of law which some years later resulted in the idea of a 'gendered law'.

The question of the nature of rape remained however a live issue during this phase. It became interconnected with issues emerging from the conflicts during the passage of the bill through Parliament and the evaluation of the results. There was no doubt that the political conflict had simplified and rigidified the reflection on sexuality, reducing it within the confines of partisan positions. On the one hand (among liberals and the left) there was the defence of 'good' sex – non-violent, egalitarian – in which a place also existed for relations between minors, and for sexual relations among handicapped and mentally disabled. On the other hand, (among Catholics and conservatives) there was the attack on sexual permissiveness as the real cause of violence.

Here, it is really possible to trace the working of two different principles: the 'left' position is in fact inspired by the principle that liberty exists in the absence of constraint, that one excludes the other and that the duty of law (of the state) is purely that of intervention in cases of proven constraint, while what must be presumed to exist in the first place is liberty (as free choice). The Catholic and conservative position subordinates the exercise of free choice to certain conditions: it is a substantivist position which not by chance can make some of the feminist arguments its own. Thus liberty cannot be presumed in the case of those who are structurally disadvantaged (minors, handicapped); the state has the duty to intervene with measures of prevention and protection: it must assume constraint on the basis of the characteristics of the actors rather than that of the actions. Liberal formalism conflicts with the casuistry of conservative substantivism, which can argue both the necessity of maintaining the presumption of violence in the case of sexual relations between minors, and that of victim-initiated proceedings in the case of spouses and cohabitees because here the primary value is not the protection of the weak but the protection of the family.

The reduction of reflections on sexuality to these two poles was what some women regarded as the worst result of the feminist campaign against sexual violence (see Bocchetti 1984). On the one hand good sex counter-posed to violence, on the other the morality of family's (good) sex counter-posed to sexual licence. The ambivalence of heterosexual relations, of love and attraction of women towards men, yet the increasingly sharp realisation that women fear men, was indicated as what prevents women from deepening their reflections on (hetero)sexuality.

> Because while in the case of abortion it was in the last analysis a matter of confrontation with the yet unborn, with those who have neither sufficient capacity nor time to win love, in the case of sexual violence it is necessary to confront and take a distance from the already existing. Here the sexual difference discourse becomes painful, threatening soli-tude and sterility. . . . Women know that a reflection on sexual violence would spread into their whole lives like a drop of ink on a piece of blotting paper, and they resist facing up to it in order to maintain a form of survival which, even though brutal, allows them to talk, join in activities, go to the cinema or just keep up their spirits in the everyday male world.
>
> (Bocchetti op. cit. p. 6)

The struggle for the law on sexual violence can thus be seen as an escape from finding oneself immersed in such an overwhelming awareness.

The supporters of the popular initiative for the law on sexual violence, for their part, while continuing to defend it as an instrument 'which has made possible the opening up throughout the country of an enormous process of growing awareness of the nature of sexuality and sexual violence' (Intervention by the sponsoring committee of the law on sexual violence 1986) themselves felt the need to propose a reflection on the nature of sexuality which distinguished itself both from the conservative outcome of the debate in parliament and from the positions of the dissi-dents, often accused of complicity with 'patriarchy'. It was in this reflec-tion that the contradictions between conceptions of sexual violence and the struggle for a change in the criminal law resurfaced most. Sexual violence was here indeed seen as sexual, rather, as the result of a violent 'phallo-cratic' heterosexuality, in which pleasure is derived from the oppression and humiliation of women. A dominant heterosexuality which with the 'sexual revolution' of the last twenty years had become even more pervasive and menacing: sexual liberty was redefined in this reflection as indiscriminate male access to the female body (see Intervention ibid.). If, however, rape is conceived as not at all a form of deviance, but on the contrary as a normal practice and the symbolic form of the sexual relations between men and women, what sense and what function can a criminal law which could only distinguish between rape and normal heterosexuality, perform? If we can never speak of free consent to sexual relations on the part of women, what could be the significance of a criminal law whose concept of crime starts precisely from the absence of consent?

The law passed by the Chamber proceeded to the justice commission of the Senate which reintroduced mandatory prosecution even in the case of sexual violence between spouses and cohabitees. In the summer of 1986 the debate in the Chamber was blocked by discussion of this amendment. The fall of the government meant that the bill also fell.

PIETÀ L'È MORTA: GENDERED LAW

A new phase opened with the new Parliament. Taking the initiative, the women elected to the Chamber on the electoral platforms of the Communist Party, the Socialist Party, the Independent Left, and the Social Democrats, drew up a bill the signatories to which included, besides some Greens, also a Christian Democrat, Maria Fida Moro. The new bill was introduced as the result of an understanding between women which cut across party lines.

The election campaign of 1986 was indeed characterised by the debate, in which feminism was involved, on the question of female political representation, after which within the Communist Party, women organised themselves around the Women's Charter (*Sezione femminile del PCI*, 1986), which highlighted the autonomy of women within the Party, the strong and privileged relation with women's and feminist issues outside the party, and launched the slogan '*Dalle donne la forza delle donne*' (from women comes the strength of women). One of the results of this was the presence of many women in leading positions in the Communist Party electoral list and an election campaign marked by the demand 'vote woman'.

Debates and polemics broke out around this understanding of the politics of women's representation (see Boccia, Peretti 1988). Some denied the possibility and the legitimacy of a 'representation of gender' in the political process while others evaluated positively the effect of a symbolic representation of sexual difference consequent upon an entry *en masse* of women into Parliament. All this however was indicative of an increased distancing from the position, dominant during the 1970s, predicating the rejection of a direct involvement with the forms and arenas of traditional politics and corresponding to the furtherance of a position in which the traditional alienation of women from the political process was recast as the basis of a project for the genderisation of the world: of a 'symbolic inscribing of sexual difference' in culture, politics and social life.

The women elected to Parliament in 1986 were 10 per cent of the total members, the highest number ever recorded. But this was not perhaps the main result of the changed political climate among women; more important in my view was the virtual annulment of the distance between the women Members of Parliament (especially those elected on the Communist Party lists) and women outside Parliament who related in various ways to the women's movement and identified themselves as feminists. The bill on sexual violence was an example of this. It was drawn up by women parliamentarians and not by this or that political party, and had as its main interlocutors women in general and those of the 'women's movement' in particular. The continuity between those who drew up the bill and the campaign outside Parliament, most importantly that which grew out of the earlier popular initiative for legal reform, was unbroken. The campaign sought to develop an understanding among women which cut across the political parties, and whereas naturally the drafters assumed final responsibility for it, the bill was presented as the putting into effect of a precise mandate conferred on the elected by the electors. This contributed to the further limitation of the autonomy and room for manoeuvre on the part of the drafters: as I have argued elsewhere (Pitch 1984), the elimination of the distance between the movement's various sites of action and the forms of political mediation and negotiation removed autonomy of initiative from both and confused the motives of one with the motives of the other. The misconception, on the part of the women Members of Parliament, that it was possible to speak on behalf of a supposedly monolithic and united women's movement imposed a rigidity every bit as strict as that of party discipline.

The proposal of the parliamentary group ran over again the fundamental points of the popular initiative for legal reform: sexual violence as a crime against the person, the reunification under a single category of crimes of carnal violence and acts of violent lust, mandatory prosecution, the introduction of the category of group rape, summary trial in open court, the possibility of civil action for compensation – subject to the agreement of the victim – by associations and movements (provided that the latter had been in existence for at least two years prior to the case) which 'have among their aims the protection of the interests injured' by the offence. Also the offence of presumed rape was to be abolished.

The Senate ended in approving a law which introduced a double standard: mandatory prosecution in all cases except those which involved spouses or cohabitees, where proceedings would be initiated by the victim. The signatories to the proposal voted against: they preferred this compromise – in which they were defeated – than to propose victim-initiated proceedings in all cases. Mandatory prosecution was thus confirmed as a fundamental question of principle by these parliamentarians just when contrary voices from women had become more numerous and authoritative.[14]

The source of many of these voices lay in the participation in the discussion of women who, after the initial polemics, had for ten years kept quiet, reluctant to acknowledge directly the appeals and the legacies of a politics which seemed to them to be purely concerned with demands (see Libreria delle donne di Milano 1987). But in ten years, as I have already pointed out, many things had changed. There was no longer, among other things, the traditional alliance between women and liberal intellectuals which had led many to be publicly sceptical of the law as an instrument and to keep a distance from anything which could be seen as a re-legitimisation of the criminal justice system, and which led all, including the promoters of the popular initiative for legal reform, to profess one's own disinterest in punishment and one's unease towards proposals of an explicitly punitive nature.

At precisely the same time as the Senate was debating the most recent bill, a left wing journalist, sent to cover a rape trial, declared his own ambivalence, his own empathy towards the defendants, guilty indeed, but nevertheless poor ignorant wretches at bottom, distorted products of a masculine and violent culture. This time response from women was immediate and unwavering: enough of these justifications and lamentations which only serve to cover up, displacing onto 'society', 'culture', the joint responsibility of all men: if it is (male) society which is violent, what well intentioned males can and ought to do is examine their own responsibility and complicity. In the meantime, as far as women are concerned, '*pietà l'è morta*' (pity is dead) (Dominijanni 1988): or, we are by now well beyond the time in which you took us for allies and subordinates in your struggles. . . .

This cool objectivity, the calmness in asserting complete autonomy of judgement proceeded from a deepening reflection which, under the banner of a 'theory of sexual difference' emphasised the priority in establishing relations, real and symbolic, within one's own gender, such as to connote one's social involvement and by which to evaluate proposals and projects as well as to produce them.

The question of mandatory prosecution was taken up again, then, to show how considerations of legal coherence and principle (the fact that mandatory prosecution applied to all 'serious' crimes, that it functioned as a public acknowledgement of such seriousness and that the offence punished was an offence against the whole community and with which the entire community was concerned) were not only extraneous to, but in contradiction to the experience and thinking of women, when they 'start from themselves' and confront themselves with, and refer themselves to other women (see Libreria delle donne di Milano, 1988 p. 1). Neither is the other consideration, that mandatory prosecution is a better protection for women inasmuch as it frees them from fear and the risk of blackmail, to be seen as more in harmony with women's needs. If, it was argued, it is true that many women are frightened of reporting crime and facing trial procedures, the wish to impose such things on them would be the act of a minority taking upon itself the role of repressive pedagogue, and thereby confirming through institutional protection, female weakness. In this case as in all others, the 'road to women's freedom' was to be seen rather in the construction of relations between women such as to 'empower' the individual woman in deciding whether or not to utilise the criminal law.

There were thus three elements to the rejection of mandatory prosecution: it is demanded by some women 'on behalf' of all women while such representativeness cannot in fact be assumed; it presupposes and confirms the weakness of women; and it conflicts with self-determination.

What this position argued for was a distancing from the existing criminal law, no longer in terms of a radical critique of, or maintaining a distance from, 'institutions', but rather from the standpoint of two interrelated objectives: the construction of normative relations between women and the foundation of a 'gendered law'.

BRIEF INSTRUCTIONS FOR THE USE OF ITALIAN FEMINIST THOUGHT

This type of argument had its roots in what in Italy is called the 'sexual difference theory'. Actually, theory is a very bad translation for 'pensiero', a word which signifies the interrelated processes of reflection upon one's political practice, and, conversely, of engaging in practice upon the basis of one's reflection. The 'theory' of sexual difference is not a theory – not only in the sense that it presupposes a practice, but also in that it does not constitute a unitary, and even less a systematic, body of concepts. Also, though the notion of sexual difference has been widely adopted throughout Italian feminism, it has been interpreted and used in different, and sometimes even contradictory ways. As here I am not trying to describe and discuss the varieties of Italian feminism, I shall only indicate what I think are the prevalent meanings of this notion, and especially those which had an impact on the way Italian feminists dealt with the issue of the law on rape at this time. Here, I only want to stress something which I think is peculiar to Italian feminist thought: by and large, and especially in its more sophisticated appearances, it is based on and refers to political practices. It is produced by these practices and in turn it produces them. Academic feminism is virtually non-existent, apart from a flourishing women's history. Italian feminist thought is political not merely because it addresses recognisably political issues (in fact, it often does not), but rather because it is never separated from some kind of political practice. The practice of sexual difference is at the same time its 'theory', or rather, what the theory and practice of sexual difference ought to produce is . . . sexual difference. Though, as I said, sexual difference has come to connote different practices, the underlying assumption is that it stands for a political practice which is characterised by the establishment of privileged real and symbolic relationships among women. It is through these relationships that each woman deals with the world, be it the everyday world of labour, that of traditional political relations (for example, within a political party or a trade union), or the world of 'culture', science, art. It is these relationships that are taken to mediate between the single woman and the rest of the world; they constitute at the same time her political practice and her source of reflection upon it and the world. A sexual difference approach does entail a 'separatist' practice, but not a separate life: in fact, it has been developed as a way to enable women to fully participate (even 'succeed') in the 'mixed' world of their choice without ceasing to be women-identified women.

I am talking here of Italian feminist *thought*: the Italian women's movement is something else, much more varied and fragmented. As I said earlier, 'movement' is not the most apt concept, evoking as it does a somewhat unitary, or at least considering itself as such, collective actor. No such thing exists any longer: there are varied feminist issues and feminist practices dislocated all through the social and political arena. Not all of them have adopted a sexual difference approach, and some of them are strongly in disagreement with its political practice. Nonetheless sexual difference is what characterises Italian feminist thought (though, I repeat, in different versions). And a sexual difference approach has been very influential in reorienting feminist politics toward the law on rape, and in opening up the issue of 'gendered law'.

The prevalent and more influential interpretations of sexual difference see it neither simply as a social and historical condition – as the result of an oppression to be overcome – nor purely as an asocial and ahistorical ontological given – and hence as invariable. It is rather seen both as an original given and as a political objective, in the sense that the original presence of two sexes is understood as having been cancelled by a history which has seen the male sex/gender impose itself as not only the dominant but the exclusive, the universal standard which has given its meaning to language, thought, and human history. The obliteration of the female gender is, in this conception, an historical event: it is a question thus, for women, of action to reaffirm, on all levels, the symbolic and social existence of two genders.

In order for this to happen, however, it is necessary first of all that women reconstitute themselves as a gender which in and for itself 'bestows value', that is, that they start to give value to their own experiences and institute relationships, horizontal and vertical, concrete and symbolic, which will allow them autonomy of evaluation and judgement, and by which they will be able to recognise authority in each other and to mediate between themselves and social reality. This would imply that the anarchy of social relations between women, when these relations are ruled by males, must be overcome: the elaboration of rules for these relations is seen as a necessary precondition to confronting the problem of rules for the relations between genders (see Diotima 1987; Irigaray 1985).

This is the context in which the idea of a gendered law is situated. Existing law is seen as providing for the existence of a single sex/gender and denying women the status of subjects, re-absorbing them into a 'neuter' individual which is easily revealed as a construction of the experiences and the interests of (certain) men, or relegating them to particular spheres, such as family or motherhood, through a protective legislation which confirms the status of women as appendices and subordinates of the male (for an analysis of the Italian criminal code which arrives at similar considerations see Virgilio 1987). The existing law, then, is one which regulates the conflicts among male interests. It cannot regulate the conflict between the sexes since the female sex is not recognised.

A gendered law, according to this conception, can at present only arise from trials and legal proceedings (Campari, Cigarini 1989), because it is there that meaningful relations between women – clients, lawyers, judges – can be established in such a way as to lead to a knowledge of the requirements and interests of women which can form the basis of an independent creation of norms. This knowledge and this practice are taken to have so far led to the elaboration of some principles which are considered essential elements of a gendered law (see Campari, Cigarini ibid.): such principles can be seen as standing in various relations to male law: of autonomy, convergence, or conflict. An example of autonomous principles would be the inscribing into law of the principle of the inviolability of the female body; an example of conflictual principle could be the legislation relating to the relations between spouses and family members; an example of a convergent principle 'can be the legislation for the repression of sexual violence'. Here in fact male law would intervene with a law 'repressing the crime to protect the orderly development of relations between citizens' (males presumably), while women's law would guarantee the inviolability of women's bodies:

> through the valorisation of the female genealogy, the responsibility of
> the mother towards her own sex, hence toward the sex of the raped

woman, the withdrawal of solidarity with the rapist son as an expression of maternal authority exercised in the name of her own sex.[15]

(Campari, Cigarini, 1989 p. 3)

Returning to the issues discussed up to this point: feminists should not get involved, according to this line of argument, in a struggle for the recognition of women as 'persons', defined as such in terms of a criminal law whose gendered nature remains hidden within the apparent neutrality of male jurisprudence, but rather they should work for the introduction as a *constitutional* principle of the right to the inviolability of the female body. Criminal law should then regain fully its real meaning and function of regulation of conflicts between men, by intervening to punish male behaviour. Women however would contribute to the re-establishment of the order threatened by sexual violence by means of rules (and presumably, practices) oriented to the strengthening of the priority of the responsibility of each woman towards all others, such as to lead to the withdrawal of support and affective relations from male rapists.

RESPONSIBILITY AND SUBJECTS

The thinking briefly summarised above seems to cut the gordian knot of the problem of whether sexual violence is sex or violence, and the associated question of the nature of consent, the extent of self-determination, the meaning of women's freedom and the political issues related to it. This is because the starting point is not the analysis of particular relations between men and women, but the postulate of women's freedom as emerging from the construction of privileged relations between women themselves. The question of consent and self-determination is displaced, or rather, becomes fluid and political. It is no longer relegated to the realm of 'natural rights', but neither is it entirely fictitious as argued by those who see consent to (and the pleasures of) heterosexuality as purely the result of domination. Rather it is intertwined with the growth, practical and symbolic, of a 'common world of women' ('common world' is a notion developed by Hannah Arendt, and refers to that public space constructed by unique, concrete, individuals confronting each other face to face: it is the realm of politics, which regains its Greek meaning of the site for the exercise of freedom and the full realisation of one's potential capabilities). Only when this common world begins to take shape, is it possible to think of a development of norms regulating the relations between it and the male world. This also means that it is on the basis of the formation of such a common world that perceptions of relations between the sexes change and the conditions of 'consent' are changed. (For a discussion of the problems which this poses for 'critical' criminology and sociology of law see Pitch 1985.)

To return to the question of sexual violence, the implication is precisely, as I have said, that of situating consent (to heterosexuality) within the changing of women's perceptions consequent on the changing of women's politics. But on another level, that of the relations between women and men, it implies the identification of consent, not as 'the bell proclaiming natural liberty' (Vega 1988 p. 84) as in the conception which separates sex from violence, nor as the sign of a total colonisation – as in the conception in which heterosexuality is itself violence, but rather as intertwined with domination, so that its interpretation and its mode of expression are relative to changes in relations between women and men, in large part today dependent on the autonomous politics of women. This politics has then to be interrogated not only with respect to the premises from which it starts out, but also with regard to its consequences.

As regards the law against sexual violence two positions met and conflicted. The first, responsible for the writing of the popular initiative for legal reform and the successive campaign, chose to use the scenario offered by the criminal law to signify in a public and dramatic form women's political presence, the seriousness of the problem under examination, and the responsibility of men for the problem. The contents of the bill (and above all the issue of mandatory prosecution) were consistent with these objectives. That meant the consideration of violence and heterosexuality as separate, distinguishable, seeing consent and coercion as mutually exclusive, removing from the act of sexual violence connotations of gender and sexuality: in a word, proceeding on the basis of a project of legal equality with men through the solemn recognition of women as legal 'persons'. The problematic nature of relations between men and women was evaded in their reduction by the criminal law to a question of violence enforced by individual men on individual women, the responsibility of men (of male society) though frequently affirmed, became concentrated in the single offender. Women's 'freedom' which would be confirmed by the principle of consent, remained, however, ahistorical and it was not by chance that the only status available to actual women was that of victim which, in the legal process, risked becoming a confirmation of passivity.

The second position, which became clear as time progressed, started from the rejection of direct legislation and focused on two proposals, seen as interconnected: prioritising legal procedures as an area in which women's needs could emerge through the mediation of relations between women (clients, lawyers, judges) and the development of practices leading to the development by women of a sense of responsibility for one another. This in turn implied the construction of a terrain in which women could choose whether or not to contend with legal procedures and together could contribute to confronting the problem of sexual violence through an interruption of the existing relations between the sexes (withdrawal of support from the son, brother, husband). As far as the content of the legislation was concerned, proceedings initiated by the defendant could only be preferred as a device which, by leaving to the individual woman the choice whether or not to report, would stimulate other women to create the conditions making it possible.

Following the first position to its extreme consequences, we might say that here mandatory prosecution (and the logic from which it derives) is seen as an instrument for the production of responsibility among men, a responsibility, however, which extends only as far as criminal indictment and denotes a referral of the consequences of *an* act to *an* actor, but which does not imply the necessity of taking responsibility for the root causes and the consequences of an act beyond those of its legal repression. As has already been said, the victims of that act are collective protagonists up to the moment in which it becomes recognised as a crime, at which point they immediately become passive, merely the grounds (in the best of cases) for the attribution of individual responsibility.

According to the second position, victim-initiated proceedings (and the logic of which they form part) are to be understood, by contrast, as an instrument for the production of responsibility among women: an assumption of responsibility which means taking on board if not the roots of violence, certainly its consequences for women, and has therefore an interactive sense, as a type of responsibility that takes care of personal relations (see Gilligan 1987). Female protagonism is here not linked to victim status and is not exhausted therefore in the recognition of a certain action as crime. It is rather connected to the imperative derived from this assumption of responsibility, and manifests itself both inside and outside the court room.

In this perspective, however, the question of the responsibility of, and the assumption of responsibility by, men, remains in the shadows, delegated on one side to the workings of the apparatus of 'male law' and on the other, to the imposition of a female authority in affective relations. 'Gendered law', in this version, does not shun criminal law but delegates it to the male. I see a risk here of merely supporting the existence of two different logics constitutive of the male and female subjects, the first entrusted to the development of a responsibility linked exclusively to the 'property' of the act, substantiated by rights which define individual liberty in 'negative' terms, the second entrusted to the development of a relational responsibility, tending towards care and obligation. That these two different logics are effectively traceable to and embodiments of different ethics, that of rights and that of responsibility, has been affirmed by some interesting research in social psychology (see again, Gilligan 1987);

however this only postpones the problem of how these two logics are able to interact and converge in such a way that the female subject is granted the freedom to enjoy rights as a woman, and that men integrate a relational responsibility into their own construction as subjects. The delegation to the criminal law of the power to settle conflicts between men risks re-establishing in another form the supposed, traditional, dichotomy between 'community' and 'society' and the different logics which are said to infuse them, without subjecting the statutory nature and function of criminal law itself to critical analysis, as they would not be of interest to women.[16]

We know moreover that up till now women have lived in a world elaborated in male terms, and so the project of 'genderising' that world cannot avoid taking into account the fact that it is precisely in a world of relations between the sexes that we live, and what we decide to avoid discussing does not thereby cease to exist and have consequences. Neither is criminal law in force only for men: the use of the legal process demonstrates that it can be useful also for women. But the opposite also holds: it is not without consequences for women what type of criminal law is in force in a particular society, and what specific body of law regulates the relations of violence between the sexes.

Finally, both positions have to confront the symbolic potential of criminal law: because while the latter, as has been argued in another chapter, may establish the innocence of the victim, it does so at the cost of confirming the abstract and universal status of the notion of victim and the construction of the victimisation as the result of an interaction between two parties rigidly separate and characterised only by the innocence (and passivity) of the one and the culpability (and activity) of the other. What space is left here to affirm and pursue sexual difference? On the other hand, are victim-initiated proceedings and an emphasis on legal procedures sufficient, without attacking the constitutional basis of criminal law itself (assuming this were possible) for a project of women's freedom distinguishable from 'consent' as conceived in the liberal political tradition and symbolically affirmed in criminal law?

The case of sexual violence seems to me particularly indicative, if nothing else, of the impossibility of 'normalisation', of the irreducibility of this crime to a crime like all others, not only from the standpoint of women – because it is, in the final analysis, a sexual and gendered crime – but also from the standpoint of criminal law itself, because it is the only crime which becomes such if it is so *named* by the victim. The question of consent is fundamental also because it is only its absence (to which only the victim can in the last analysis testify) which renders this crime a crime. We know how much ambiguity there is in this consent, and that it must be understood and situated in a context of power. However, when consent is inscribed into the criminal law, it loses its ambiguity, with, in addition to the symbolic effects, the practical consequence of allowing in fact a trial of the victim, the only person who is able to say whether a crime took place. There are possible correctives to this process[17] but it cannot avoid remaining central.

LESS LAW

In 1989 a new code of penal procedure was introduced. Italian criminal proceedings changed from inquisitorial to (more or less) adversarial. Some of the provisions contained in the bill were thereby rendered obsolete (summary trial, the constitution of associations for civil redress; the introduction of plea bargaining and changes in the role of the offended party).

At this point, even the most staunch feminist supporters of the bill presented by the women parliamentarians conceded that a revision of their position was in order. Doubts concerning not only the law against rape but also the use of legal instruments to achieve women's freedom became more widespread.

Our present Parliament (elected on 5 April 1992) is very different from past Parliaments: the Communist Party dissolved, and its successor (PDS, the Democratic party of the Left) gained only 17 per cent of the votes; right wing formations increased their constituencies and votes; old alliances are difficult, new ones at present impossible. So far, the rape bill has not been put on the agenda for discussion. Those women on the left who have been re-elected chose not to press for a speedy discussion, for two interconnected reasons. On the one hand, many of them have come to share the feminist critiques of the bill; on the other hand they fear that the Catholic forces, by now the more interested in the approval of a rape bill, will further distort its meaning and contents.

For, as in the case of prostitution, legislating against rape offers the occasion to pass repressive laws on sexual behaviour and to generally express a repressive sexual culture. As we have seen, such occasions have been seized many times during the history of rape bills, in the name of the protection of the weak and disabled (statutory rape in case of sexual intercourse with and between minors and mentally handicapped people), or of the sacredness of the family (the double standard, i.e. mandatory prosecution in case of all rapes except those occurring between spouses and cohabitees).

Again the question arises, whether it is possible to legislate on sexuality and sexual relations without being caught in the trap of censoring sexuality and sexual relations. Laws dealing with sexuality cannot be 'liberating'. I do not mean to say that some form of 'authentic' sexuality exists, and that law and other discourses necessarily 'discipline' and censor it. Law, medicine, culture contribute to the construction of the sexuality we know (see Foucault 1976): yet, law, medicine, culture are male (among other things), that is, permeated by gender relations. As these relations change, there is the possibility that other forms of sexuality and sexual relations develop and affirm themselves. Certainly, the feminist struggles to change rape laws arose from and tried to affirm new sexual relations. Yet, concentrating on legal change did not help this process of development, construction and affirmation. More importantly, the drawbacks and backlashes of such struggles should not be seen only as the results of defeats, difficult compromises, a resistant masculinist culture and society. The most that law can do is register the actual state of *gender* relations: when it is referred to in order to establish the confines between good and bad sex – as a law on rape cannot escape doing – then it forecloses the possibility of further elaboration on sexuality and it opens the way to a widening of the sphere of 'bad sex'.

Throughout Western Europe rape laws have been amended or proposals for amendments have been discussed in the past twenty years along similar lines. The results are laws, or proposals, that combine the 'normalisation' of rape with an extension of the sphere of bad sex. Rape is defined as a crime against persons, whose authors and victims may be both men and women; anachronistic 'protective' norms (seduction) are abolished; distinction between rape 'proper' and other violent sexual acts is usually abolished; the area of 'presumed rape' (statutory rape) is widened; new sexual crimes are introduced (laws on pornography, for example). Paradoxically, though explicit references to women disappear, what we have are laws which once again construct women's sexuality (and women as such) as in need of protection, similar in this to children and the mentally handicapped. But it is precisely the disappearance of gendered actors as authors and victims that facilitates this outcome. These norms are in principle designed to defend anybody's 'sexual freedom', by threats that might come from anybody: then, there follows a series of norms designed to protect 'the weak' from coercive sex, where coercion is presumed precisely on the basis of the 'weakness' of supposed victims. Since it is men who rape and since they rape women (or, occasionally, other men, thereby 'reduced' to a feminine position), the 'sexual freedom' that is defended is women's, thereby made analogous to the 'sexual freedom' of those presumed never to be free to 'consent'.

Yet, of course, the question of rape must be confronted, and it must be confronted also on the legal level, at the very least for its symbolic value. But it must be confronted by keeping well in mind what it implies, e.g. legislating about sexuality, an act of censorship rather than an act of and for freedom. Thus, we may decide that less is better: or, that we'd be better off with as 'light' a law as possible.

Not even the best possible rape law can sanction or signify women's freedom, nor represent the standard by which to measure gender and sexual relations. We should be content with a law that is the least offensive to women, but which is 'light' enough not to involve us in repressive legislation on sexuality, and even less in curbing women's freedom. The less detailed such a law the better; the more spaces it leaves for women's initiatives the better, including, of course, victim-initiated proceedings in all cases.

Perhaps we should start to reflect on rape by relating it to the questions of abortion and reproductive technologies, rather than to those of other 'sexual' crimes. There are risks in this strategy, namely those of reconceiving the female gender primarily in reproductive terms. But I believe that the gains are greater.

Rape, the criminalisation of abortion (and, in different ways, its legalisation), the actual development of reproductive technologies and of the laws that are being discussed to discipline them all have to do with women's lack of full sovereignty over their own bodies. It is sovereignty that we must gain, sovereignty that must be recognised. The proposal to think in terms of a constitutional principle stating the inviolability of women's bodies, though it displaces rape from its usual site within 'sexual' crimes, merely states a negative freedom. Women's sovereignty, on the other hand, implies power, the positive freedom to do and act. It is this sovereignty that rape threatens, and rape (and abortion) laws limit, fail to recognise, put under protection. As to laws on reproductive technologies, designed apparently to curb the discretionary power of doctors, they in fact tend to heavily limit women's knowledge of and access to them. Both in the case of abortion and of reproductive technologies, the recourse to 'ethics' (bio-ethical committees are being set up everywhere, and they are the strongest source of new legislation) is the newest means to deny women's full control (and full responsibility) over their own bodies.

This recourse to ethics is deployed, by those in search of a non-religious ethics, in the language of rights. Women's rights are set against the rights of potential fathers, embryos and foetuses. That is why, among other things, simply fighting for a *right* to self-determination is not only insufficient, but also misleading.

A politics of sovereignty would displace law from its central place in discourse, reflection and conflict and would challenge rights rhetoric and policies by confronting them with the self-constitution of a concrete, embedded, subject. A politics of sovereignty would imply empowering practices rather than demands for more, new, protective legislation.

Perhaps, such politics might imply both using to our advantage existing laws, without trying to get new ones, and deconstructing, rendering symbolically and practically meaningless, those we cannot use to our advantage. Perhaps, such politics implies less, rather than more, law. When Italian feminists started fighting around the abortion issue, they asked for a law assuring that abortion would be free, available on demand and safe. Today, fourteen years after the law was passed, many feminists would agree that decriminalisation, i.e., the disappearance of abortion from the legal codes, would be preferable. Abortion constitutes the only example of the inclusion of a gendered principle (of the kind we are struggling for) in legislation: its cancellation from legal codes would sanction women's power (and responsibility) not only over (for) their own bodies but over (for) the whole sphere of reproduction. The law does embody this principle, but makes it subject to scrutiny by the rest of society and its representatives, medical doctors. When it was asked for (feminists *campaigned* for the legalisation of abortion, but did not write their own bill), not only cultural and political conditions appeared extremely unfavourable to simple de-criminalisation (they are still – perhaps more – unfavourable), but the idea of women's individual and collective strength, of a female freedom which need not wait for the complete defeat of social and economic oppression, was still undeveloped. *More* law seemed necessary to curb the arbitrary power of men; though the State's intervention into so-defined private matters was always seen with suspicion, and ambivalence, both theo-retically and in practice, was maintained towards it. The idea was still prevalent that a number of new laws (in the sphere of work as in that of the family and regarding abortion and rape) was, if not sufficient, necessary to women's freedom.

During the years many such laws were demanded and some of them were passed. The struggle around rape, however, and the implementation of the abortion law, made more evident that, though legal changes may be useful, in certain cases absolutely necessary, they are not only always ambiguous and prone to different interpretations, but also they do not, by themselves, either foster or produce freedom. Some even claimed that the legalisation of abortion had in some way contributed to the dissolution of that female solidarity which had helped many women to get abortions when it was still illegal. Without going to such extremes, certainly the abortion law, while it was a great progress, still subjects women to the scrutiny of doctors in particular (who increasingly refuse to perform abortions on the grounds of conscientious objection) and of society in general. The very existence of such a law supports a culture which refuses women sovereignty over their own bodies and thereby fosters distrust over their ability to assume responsibility for themselves, their partners, society, the human species.

The postulate of women's freedom, to be acted upon and recognised through 'faithfulness to one's own sex', may help in adopting a different attitude towards the law. An attitude which is more flexible, which privileges using the law rather than producing it – as in the case of the establishment of relationships between women clients, lawyers and judges in rape trial proceedings; or, when production is inevitable, which aims for 'light' laws, that do not foreclose autonomous normative production and the self-determined development of social relations.

This might be seen to go in the direction of what some call 'reflexive law' (see Teubner 1993), of a law that confines itself to the production of a procedural frame, to be filled of content by the actors concerned themselves. Yet, 'reflexive law' would seem to leave much more space for power games within society and between society and the State that we might want to concede.

What I want to say is that I, at least, am not yet prepared to confront, let alone develop, an overall theoretical model for a 'gendered law'. It is very possible that in certain cases we may need extremely precise substantive legislation, and in other cases general procedural norms, or even no norms at all. The gendering of law has more to do with a politics of and for women's sovereignty as (individual) women than with specific pieces of legislation or the development of a general theoretical model of law. This may be considered an evasion of difficult questions. In the last chapter I shall try to argue for this position while summarising the various themes of the book.

9   A politics of sovereignty

EQUALITY, DIFFERENCE AND CRIMINAL LAW

The contemporary debate on equality – formal and substantive, simple and 'complex' – has to take into account not only the familiar problem of the relationship between protection and self-determination, but also the fact that ever new 'differences' are today reclaiming recognition as 'differences'. It is well known that the achievement of formal equality, through the fertile terrain of claims and conflicts, often produces new forms of discrimination. One of the central themes of feminist thinking was precisely that of how to escape the alternative between equality as the forced assimilation to a standard which, while neutral in appearance, is in reality defined in terms of the male gendered (as well as white, property owning, etc.) subject, and a recognition of 'difference' implying protection and discrimination. The genderisation of the legal subject (of the symbolic, of culture in general) is one attempt to find a way out of this entanglement. How to translate it, however, into a concrete politics is anything but a simple question. Whether it is in fact possible in the case of the politics of criminal justice is what I want to look at now.

The tensions which currently permeate the legal and political, as well as the philosophical, dimensions of equality are highly visible in the debate around the politics of crime. In this area, as in the more heavily scrutinised areas of welfare and employment, the relation between so-called formal equality and substantive inequalities often takes the form of a conflict between demands for the recognition of one's status as a full subject (thus requiring those legal safeguards accorded to such subjects) and demands for the recognition of one's status as a particular subject (thus requiring a differential treatment, which may take the form of either positive or negative discrimination). It is within this alternative that the issues of juvenile justice and of the mentally ill which have already been discussed are usually interpreted.

The literature on the relationship between women and criminal justice (for a bibliography see Pitch 1987) is by now substantial. While it documents the way in which legal decisions in accordance with the principles of formal equality, reinforce a differential treatment of women confirming their minority condition, it has difficulty in avoiding the alternation between, on the one hand, demands for 'full' equality and on the other, demands for the legal recognition of difference and diversity. The reason for this alternation is the fact that the same diversity is the starting point not only for negative discrimination but also at times positive discrimination.

Such an alternative is not different from those posed for other subjects defined as 'weak' (minors, the sick, etc.). In the same way as with these latter, the demand for full recognition of the actual status of 'persons' can become in practice (as in other well-known situations) a worsening of the real situation as regards court proceedings and sentencing.

As Hilary Allen (1988) points out, it is sexual difference that serves as the reference point when arguing the rationality of taking account of 'differences' of age, culture or social conditions. What this means is that sexual difference is interpreted as a difference of condition, an inequality to be either eliminated by remedial measures and redistributive policies such as positive discrimination, or to be preserved through measures of protection. Such measures pose problems in respect of the nature of the equality upon which law's neutral subject is constructed, because the latter implies the treatment of persons who are obviously different as if they were equivalent.[1] Various solutions to this dilemma have been proposed in the area of social policy. Such strategies include, as it is well known, a reinterpretation of equality as equality of opportunity; as reverse discrimination in order to compensate for past injustices; as equality of outcomes; as complex equality (theories of justice abound: for an Italian discussion, see Vega 1982; De Leonardis 1990). These strategies produce tensions and conflicts with respect to an equality defined as the irrelevance of personal differences in the enjoyment of civil rights, and in addition raise problems concerning the choice of which types of inequalities to privilege. It is not by chance, as the debates on policies directly involving women demonstrate (see Luker 1984 and AA.VV. 1986–87), that such measures generate tensions which sometimes mobilise new demands for traditional policies of protection. There is no doubt however, that the result is the confirmation of differences as inequalities, both in the enjoyment of civil rights and in access to and use of social rights (Minow 1990).

Looking at this nexus of questions through the lenses of sexual difference, rather than looking at sexual difference through the lenses of other 'differences', may offer new insights. We discover, for example, that the tensions and conflicts between civil and social rights can be understood in a new way if viewed from the standpoint of the role of the private sphere in legitimising and facilitating the enjoyment of civil and political rights (Saraceno 1988). Political citizenship ignores differences relegated to the private sphere, and only those who can either avoid the interference of such differences or succeed in making them count as general interests are truly citizens. Hence the absence of civil rights for the poor, the recipients of various types of state welfare, the insane, minors and increasingly today the tensions deriving from demands for the extension of rights also to these groups. The standpoint of sexual difference points out how these tensions have a lot to do with the construction of the citizen as a subject abstracted from attachments, responsibilities, ties (Saraceno ibid.): but also how this construction has been made possible through the assumption of the male as the neutral-universal, where the female comes to signify difference, particularity, ties, relations – all relegated to the private sphere.

The point seems to be then not so much, or not only, the extension of civil rights to the realm of the social, as much as contemporaneously the deconstruction of the subject of these rights itself. The genderisation of the subject is the precondition for the bonds, the links, the responsibility which gives substance to the concrete individual to enter into his or her constitution and for equality to develop as the recognition of, and dependence upon, difference.

This is an operation which seems certainly more practicable on the level of social policies than on that of criminal justice policies for at least two rather simple reasons. Firstly, it requires a flexible politics, conscious of the provisional and flexible nature of choices, continuously deployed in the deconstruction of the ever-present antithesis between equality and difference, tending to avoid construction of the resultant political choices in dichotomous terms. Criminal justice is an area scarcely adapted to this type of practice, not only because of what has been said above, but also on the level of normative innovation where the demand for elasticity conflicts with the principles of due process which are the only protection against the discretional use of the power to punish. If, in general, it is beneficial to move in the direction of a diminution in the role of the criminal justice system itself (see the arguments of the preceding chapters), it is rather at the frontier between criminal justice and social policy that the strategy of reintroducing, as well as recognising, differences can be located.

The symbolic power of criminal law, it has also been seen, can be utilised only by remaining within the boundaries of the criminal justice system itself, at the cost of the recognition of one's status as that of 'neutral' citizen. This can be too high a price to pay, both for the bearers of 'difference' and for female sexual difference. In the case of the former this is because if such recognition is not accompanied by a contraction of the sphere of criminal justice and by adequate social policies, there is a risk of worsening the conditions of the 'differents' with regard to legal proceedings and sanctions. In the latter case it is (also) because female sexual difference concretised in terms of inequality, becomes simply (formally) annulled.

Nonetheless, the question of a law construed with regard to a gendered subject could have strong implications for law and the criminal justice system. It would allow the possibility of rethinking the questions of social order, social control, the disciplining of personal and social relations, from the point of view of a subject constituted by attachments and embedded in a web of relations. This would enable the emergence of a conception of responsibility construed both as an appeal for autonomy and as arising out of the interaction of these relations themselves: simultaneously and inseparably a mode of subjectivisation and expression and a mode of interdependence. With what gains, from the standpoint of the questions discussed in this book, it is easy to imagine.

FOR A POLITICS OF SOVEREIGNTY

Minors, the mentally sick, women. I have so far dealt with these three 'groups' in their encounters with criminal justice, but others may be (and have been) added: ethnic minorities, the very poor, the physically handicapped (or differently endowed) people. The list can and does go on forever, as ever new 'differences' are reclaimed in order to obtain resources or to legitimise a strongly held identity.

Women have so far generally been seen as one of these 'differences' and have been subsumed under the same arguments.

From the point of view of their relation with the law and legal discourse, they do have something in common. It is the critique of the law as using as its standard an abstract, neutral, independent and self-sufficient individual.

But 'women' are neither an oppressed nor an interest group. Nor are they a 'group'. In the very real, though merely empirical, sense that not all women are in the same position towards power, authority, wealth, and that they do not share all the same 'interests'. Neither are they comparable to ethnic minorities, as the identity they reclaim is not an ascribed one; they do not share a common culture, certainly not in the strong anthropological sense that ethnic minorities do or say they do. A woman may be rich, educated, black, sick, a child, just as a man may be rich, educated, black, sick, a child. Yet (the adult, healthy, presumably white) man is the standard by which (even the adult, healthy, white) woman is measured. Woman is not a subject in the same way man is, the human original division into two genders goes unrecognised, both symbolically, legally, and in practice. This does entail 'oppression', in certain cases the sharing of interests and even of some cultural aspects, but this does not make women analogous to other oppressed, to other interest groups or to ethnic minorities, though at some points they may share the same objectives and engage in the same struggles.

The feminist critique of the subject of rights, and of legal discourse in general, as being only apparently neutral, abstract and self-sufficient but in fact predicated on a particular construction of masculinity, is at the basis of the critique of the equality principle and equality policies insofar as they imply assimilation. In order to enjoy the same rights as an individual, it is necessary to become like them (or: there is only one way towards the achievement of the status of individual). But there is a more important aspect to this critique, and that is precisely the questioning of freedom as the property of an individual without ties and relationships. The feminist reclaiming of difference is thus not one more specification of the standard subject, but rather signifies the attempt at the construction of a subject whose freedom is a function of relationships, whose freedom is not diminished by them (by what makes each of us what each of us is), but on the contrary it gains sense, meaning, direction by them. It is precisely the relationship between freedom and responsibility, the fact that independence is a function of dependence, that self-sufficiency is never a given, but rather the ability to negotiate relationships, to assume responsibility for them, to acknowledge one's dependence on them that I consider to be at the core of the feminist reflection and practices on law and politics.

I should like to name the politics that are suggested by this approach to individual freedom (autonomy, self-determination) the politics of sovereignty. This politics stands in contrast to a politics of identity, which I see as denoting methods of demanding, and contents of demands predicated on the assumption of an already-existing, ascribed, 'identity', be it a cultural, social, or biological one. The multiplication and specification of rights are a consequence of such a politics. On the one hand, it risks being merely declamatory, on the other to submerge individual rights within group rights, as it reaffirms the primacy of ascribed characteristics in designating membership in the group.

Some of the actors I described in chapter 4 may be seen as engaging in a politics of sovereignty. Mothers of drug addicts, victims of the Mafia, relatives of the mentally ill, victims of terrorism have at least this in common (however we may evaluate what they ask for): they are citizens who gather to act publicly on questions that interest them personally, as individual members of families.

They testify to an assumption of responsibility *vis-à-vis* each other and, through each other, to the whole society, for the production, management and solution of problems which otherwise would either remain private or be delegated to institutional care. A culture of rights is here reinterpreted as a culture of mutual responsibilities. People confront each other, and choose each other, 'heavy' with what each of them is, but this 'heaviness' is used as a resource rather than as an impediment to action. The group is not based on a pre-set identity and it does not confer one. There is no free-riding: indeed, the main 'objective' of the group is the existence of and participation into the group itself, as what is promoted or fought for has closely to do with each individual's sense of self, dignity, autonomy (Turnaturi 1991). Action and objective of the action coincide: it is by the fact that I personally act, that I assume responsibility myself for what I am and want to be, that I can recognise myself as fully a citizen. This recognition is public in two senses: because it is mediated by others who act in the same way, and because by this very collective action a public sphere is created. Such public sphere is political in the sense that Hannah Arendt (1989) gives to this notion; it is the sphere created by the actions of concrete, different individuals coming face to face, related by their choosing to act together, yet separate because unique.

Women's politics, as it is based upon practices and produces theories attempting to combine freedom and responsibility, is a politics of sovereignty. It aims to realise 'the human condition of a plurality of unique beings' (Cavarero 1992), whose first form is 'the duality of being man and being woman'. To reclaim this duality from biology, necessity, means to conceive it as implying action, politics. In this sense

> women's belonging to the female gender constructs the public space of gendered action, and the relationship between women is this action. It is action, i.e. freedom, because the gendered determination of being is no more destiny, nature, but condition of possibility. . . . Gender mediates between singularity and plurality, between the irreducibility of the self and the common world that unites and separates one self from the other.
>
> (Boccia 1989)

To take seriously a politics of sovereignty means, I think, to abandon the very idea of a search for a coherent, all-encompassing model for political action, on the one hand, and for institutional transformation on the other: both from the point of view of the collective actors engaging in such a politics and from the point of view of those who try to devise institutional answers to accommodate such a politics.

A politics of sovereignty is better understood within a paradigm that privileges a processual rationality: this paradigm permits the accommodation of diverse approaches, without pretending to reduce them to a synthesis. From the point of view of actors, for example, the relationship with institutions may be characterised by a conflictual-collaborating stance (mothers of drug-addicts, relatives of the mentally ill), by an 'opportunistic' use of existing laws and of existing institutional spaces (women), by attitudes favourable to de-legalisation (women again), or, on the contrary, by attempts more rigorously to determine specific competences and duties (as in the case of institutional actors such as social workers). I see the project of 'gendering' law within such a politics of sovereignty. I do not think only that the construction of a general theoretical model is premature, I think that to go looking for it would be contrary to the logics of a politics of sovereignty.

This whole book argues (I do not know how successfully) for an approach that privileges process over structure, flexibility and reversibility to global planning, taking seriously and learning from consequences to imputing 'perverse' consequences to mistakes, evil intentions, inadequate planning. This approach, though critical of current rights policies and discourses (as I tried to argue both in the case of minors and women) insofar as they privilege an abstract freedom and exclude the assumption and attribution of responsibility, should nonetheless remain open to the possibility of a reformulation of these policies. Restoring civil rights to the mentally ill was at the same time the result and the starting point of de-institutionalisation processes which challenged traditional arrangements and redistributed and rendered more complex issues of responsibility. The current crisis of welfare policies and ideologies cannot be met by reverting to liberal policies and ideologies. On the contrary, the culture of social rights that welfare has produced should be taken seriously. It is a culture which is at the basis of the protagonism and activism of many groups today, who challenge the institutions of welfare to make them accountable for the promises they did not keep. At the same time, these groups give a new meaning to citizenship, by assuming responsibility themselves towards their own welfare.

Women's politics, which is geared to the reconstitution of a political subjectivity on the basis of an embedded subject, responsible towards oneself and others, suggests looking for policies that enhance, rather than depress, the activities of *individuals*, who become individuals precisely on the basis of their relationships with others.[2]

Notes

PROCESSES AND PRODUCTS OF SOCIAL CONTROL

1 It is the difficulties inherent in the concepts of 'universal interest' and 'general consensus' which have contributed, in the North American tradition, to depriving the category of social control of its critical connotations and have conferred on it a role almost exclusively descriptive of processes associated with the production and reproduction of consensus. But its translation into micro-sociological terms (the processes of induction of actors into conformity with social norms) has to do also with the difficulty of an unambiguous identification of 'public authority' together with the problems associated with the establishment of hierarchical relations between agencies differently situated within the subsystems of society in general. (See also Fine 1987 and on the question of the relation between disorder and control see Marconi 1979.)

2 For a bibliography on ethnomethodological and phenomenological sociology see Giglioli, Dal Lago 1983; Pitch 1982.

3 If the articulation of social control in terms of therapy is situated in a political and cultural context characterised by the full development of the welfare state there is a precedent for it which I would characterise as 'Rooseveltian' (see Merton 1972 Part II chapters VI and VII) in which social control identifies rather the mechanisms of tension management between 'social structure' and 'cultural structure'. In both (Parsonian and Mertonian) versions of structural functionalism social control is first and foremost the producer of motivations to action. But in Merton's treatment this does not exclude coercive aspects and it is this version which is the more utilised by the sociology of deviance.

4 The functionalist perspective has been taken up by two different traditions. The first, the sociology of deviance, has emphasised those aspects relative to the relation between actor and system, construed as the relationship between individual and society. The second tradition has concerned itself rather with the systemic dimension, with the problem of a hierarchical ordering of norms in a situation of role differentiation. If deviance is a result of the lack of motivational links to consensual values, role differentiation does not of itself originate the conflicts which produce deviance, and therefore those values are also regulators and harmonisers of roles. Here, social control designates all the mechanisms of intra- and inter-systemic integration which contribute to the stabilisation of a hierarchy of norms. One such mechanism is law and it is above all the sociologists of law who have followed this direction. Such a

development is particularly relevant in Luhmann, see Bredemeier 1962; Friedman 1975; Luhmann 1977, 1978; Parsons 1962; and for the Italian debate see among others, De Nardis 1988; Febbrajo 1975; Ferrari 1980; Ferrari 1987; Martinelli 1988; Tomeo 1981; Treves 1987.

5 If law can in fact be seen as a mechanism of social control, it is such rather in its function of 'interpretation' and stabilisation of social norms than in the distribution of sanctions.

6 In Ross law already performs a function of this type. For the relation between this approach and the influential sociological school of jurisprudence see White 1956.

7 Where criminal law can in fact be interpreted as the main guarantor of fundamental liberties, the criminal justice system in its role as distributor of punishments and selector of individuals to undergo punishment lends itself more readily to an interpretation in terms of censure and repression.

8 This is different from the meaning of discipline as found in Foucault (1976) who uses it to underline the productivity of 'power'. Discourses and disciplinary practices are not exhausted by the state and its apparatuses but act at all levels of the social which are constituted simultaneously as the object of knowledge and the target of specific disciplinary practices. Also for Foucault discipline does not emanate from a centre, does not have a subject and is not understandable in terms of censure, even though its interpretation by sociologists of deviance and so-called critical criminologists of the 1970s has shifted it in this direction.

9 There is also the area studied elsewhere under the category of informal justice, in particular the independent and private systems of surveillance and control. These range from private police forces, the systems of control and self control of large companies, to the studies by the legal pluralists of the internal mechanisms of justice and discipline in particular organisations such as the professions or the military. See R.L. Abel 1982; Cain 1985; Olgiati, Astori 1988; Shearing, Stenning 1985; Scraton, South 1984; Spector 1981.

10 This area is the terrain of, not only so-called moral crusades, but also self-organisation to confront common problems (e.g. Alcoholics Anonymous). Many associations act both on the level of immediate politics and on the level of relations with welfare agencies and through self help groups (such as relatives of drug dependants, mentally ill etc.)

11 In Italy, discourses and projects of de-institutionalisation coincided – as has been noted – one as the motor of the other, with the wave of anti-authoritarianism symbolised by 1968 (Pitch 1982, Introduction). The debate focused particularly around law and psychiatry. There being no autonomous sociological vocabulary from which to draw concepts and analyses, the Anglo-Saxon literature was pillaged to provide a language for political projects which oscillated between 'revolutionary' maximalism and a 'modernising' reformism. The nearly contemporaneous law and order campaigns and the promulgation of emergency legislation gave rise to a debate in which the defence of civil rights and due process clashed with strong substantialist tendencies appealing both to issues of security and to the ideology of rehabilitation, formulated, for example in the Italian penal reforms of the 1980s, (see the Gozzini law of 1986) as the flexibility of punishment in response to the needs of the individual.

12 Proposals and projects of de-legalisation, the development of forms of conflict resolution outside the criminal justice system aimed at increasing the direct

participation of citizens and removing the long formal legal procedures which supposedly alienate many from claiming their rights, do not seem to have avoided similar results. This is especially true as far as the culturally disadvantaged groups and social strata are concerned. (See Abel 1979, 1982. A critique of the thesis of the extension of disciplinary control can be found in Bottoms 1983.)

13 The Italian prison reforms of 1975 and 1986, for example, introduced differentiation between dangerous and rehabilitable prisoners. The first are denied access to the benefits and sentence reductions enjoyed by the latter, and are to be subjected to a 'special regime'. Italian prison reforms suffer from a pronounced oscillatory movement in the general political climate, which strongly influences whether or not, and to what extent, they are implemented. Their logic, however, is inspired by 're-education', premised on differentiation between the re-educable and the socially dangerous (see Di Lazzaro 1988; Mosconi, Pavarini 1988).

14 On the criticism of the notion of 'success' of the reforms on the basis of a comparison with their acknowledged objectives see Cohen 1988, and more generally, Donolo, Fichera 1988.

15 Liberal and 'back to justice' models enter into this reading. One can trace similar evaluative elements in the taking up again of formalism as a form of guaranteeism in Italy. For more detail see the next chapter.

STUDYING THE 'CRIMINAL QUESTION'

1 The discussion on the 'success' of reforms, on the relations between policies and their implementation, goals and consequences, the logic of institutions and the actions of professionals, has given rise to a literature too rich and diverse to be cited here. I limit myself to indicating two recent texts, Donolo and Fichera (1988) – and the ample bibliography contained therein – and Douglas (1986). This discussion, as far as it concerns the prison and the criminal justice system and the policies which involve them, is as old as the prison itself, as Foucault observes. On the various interpretations of the 'failure' of the prison and reforms which have been concerned with it from the beginning, see Cohen and Scull eds. 1983 (esp. chapter 1).

2 Already in Durkheim (1963) the social normality of crime is argued, in polemic with Garofalo, and in general with the Italian positivist school: even if the status of normality of the individual criminal still remains ambiguous.

3 The use of the masculine pronoun here is in this case deliberate. On the empirical level, as well as on that of the studies, the criminal is male (besides being young, poor, often black). On the relation between stereotypes of the criminal and selective activities of the agencies of criminal justice see Chapman 1971.

4 In the sense that Merton, and in his wake, the greater part of American sociologists of deviance attribute to this concept: the result of a bad integration between the system of goals and norms and social structure (for a discussion and a bibliography on this concept and its use among the sociologists of deviance see Pitch 1982).

5 Of which the proposals, the prospects, the politics of de-institutionalisation, decentralisation of control, de-legalisation, territorialisation are discussed by Cohen 1983. Out of a critique of professional social work with its orientation

towards therapy and care grew the experiences and projects of community work: for a discussion see Bailey and Brake 1975.

6 Different, at least in part, is the situation in France, where the theoretical debate is strongly influenced by the work of Foucault. See however the journal *Déviance et Société* founded in 1976 and connected, at least initially, with the tendencies oriented to critical criminology and critical sociology of law.

7 Cohen (1988) distinguishes two currents. The first is that inspired by traditional conservatism which emphasises the supremacy of law and order and calls for the reinforcement of criminal justice institutions based on the idea that crime is caused by a lack of authority and that punishment serves as a deterrent. The second 'managerial' current legitimises repressive policies in terms of an ideology of efficiency and results. Both currents of the 'right' are, on the other hand, according to Cohen, nothing more than articulations of the liberal model which underlies the dominant orientations in the study and management of the issue of crime.

8 The return of mandatory sentences and fixed punishments, is argued for by the American Friends Service Committee against the 'correctional' system of which the indeterminate sentence is an instrument and a symbol. A brief discussion of the 'correctional model' in the United States can be found in Pavarini (1983); an analysis of the 'co-option' of the civil libertarian project of return to the determinate sentence by neo-conservative arguments and policies can be found in Greenberg and Humphries (1981).

9 Even if there is no shortage of theories which still link criminality to some aspects of 'human nature' be it the 'double X' chromosome, abnormal aggressive tendencies or such like.

10 There is however also an American version. See for example the issues of the journal *Crime and Social Justice* Nos. 18, 1982 and 19, 1983 dedicated to a revision of critical criminology in a 'realist' direction.

11 The demands of these groups, among others, will be different if articulated by organised groups as opposed to gathered by the sociologist through individually distributed questionnaires or deduced from bar room gossip rather than from concrete attitudes towards 'criminals'. There are not only differences which result from the mode of inquiry, but differences resulting from opinions which change depending on context and circumstances. The problematic nature of opinion surveys and their inadequacy in revealing the 'popular' will are noted by, among others, Baratta 1985 p. 451.

12 I shall return to this in the next chapter. It is evident, however, that the status of victim is not a natural condition, or, to put it better, it does not inhere in every distress but is a status ascribed or assumed, which carries a certain self-perception and a certain interpretation of the 'victimising' situation. To be a victim implies the acting out of a role, with expectations both of those who become so defined and those who define someone as a victim. It is clear that this process of definition can be, and often is, the object of negotiation and conflict, and neither is it indifferent to who defines who and to what purpose (see Miers 1983).

13 It is at least curious, for example, that on the question of prostitution we arrive at the proposal to criminalise the client in the name of both those who consider prostitution a crime against women (including in this respect a strong current of Anglo-Saxon feminism), and of those (presumably the working class) who consider it a social problem, a hidden source of degradation to the quality of life in their communities. See Box-Grainger, 1986.

RADICAL ENQUIRIES, UNFOUNDED POLICIES

1 Or rather, the law. During the 1960s a conspicuous number of lawyers and progressive judges was moved to adopt a critical position because of dissatisfaction with a law and legal philosophy whose formalism was seen as the instrument of conservatism and social injustice.

2 The birth of a true sociology of law in Italy came about with a series of research projects on the administration of justice, sponsored by the *Centro Nazionale di Prevenzione e Difesa Sociale* in 1962. The publication was introduced, discussed and summarised by Treves 1972.

3 The reference here is to the journal *La Questione Criminale*, which began in 1975, gathering together lawyers, sociologists, historians of law. This journal had its ups and downs and certainly did not express a unique theoretical and political orientation. I have recounted these events in Pitch 1983, revealing the oscillations between strong and weak anti-formalist tendencies which permeated in various forms the legal and sociological components.

4 It is the contradiction, already discussed in Foucault 1976 (see also, Melossi and Pavarini 1976) between a system of punishment oriented to retributivism and its necessary expression, the prison, which cannot but be inclined, from the outset, to correctionalist ends. For a discussion of 'useful punishment' see Pavarini 1983. An analysis of the doctrines, ideologies and theories of punishment is provided by Ferrajoli 1985, 1989.

5 The only aspect of terrorism that Italian critical criminology was able to grapple with was the analysis of emergency legislation. Particular political factors such as the adherence of the old left, having entered into the arena of government, to a politics of law and order, served to indicate on one hand the contradictions of the theoretical–ideological model deployed by this criminology (see Ferrajoli and Zolo 1977; 1978) and on the other the difficulty, intrinsic to this model, of settling accounts with types of illegality not reducible to the circular dynamic of socio-economic contradictions and institutional reaction.

6 I refer, for example, to the concept of minimal criminal law, discussed below.

7 A current of critical criminology, predominantly American, during the 1970s argued for a reversal of criminal law and justice, which were seen as focusing on the weak and defending the powerful, by defining crime as the activities, or rather their results, of the powerful themselves: imperialism, capitalism, exploitation, racism etc. (see Platt 1973; Schwendinger and Schwendinger 1973).

8 See for example the polemic of Matza (1976) against the 'correctionalist' attitude of the sociologist of deviance, who thereby embraces the aims of the agencies of control and denies herself the possibility of 'understanding' the phenomenon under investigation.

9 Not in the sense which ethnology traditionally attributes to it of an observer who sheds her mental clothing, system of values, in order to enter as far as possible into sympathy with the observed culture, intending however not to 'contaminate' it with their presence. The meaning is more that of an observer who contributes with her analysis to change the problem and naturally partakes of responsibility for it.

10 These three phenomena are examples of informal justice even if not of the type invoked by 'the left'. See on this theme, the bibliography in the note to the preceding chapter.

11   The fact that this crisis gives rise to this particular form of self-organisation rather than the creation of autonomous social service agencies, or that contemporary vigilantism does not seem to be connected, as in the past (remember Malcolm X!) to other projects in or for the community, is a question of considerable relevance. If vigilantism seems to allude to an attempt at the 'reappropriation' of direct control over conditions of life, to direct assumption of responsibility, it appears also, however, to cohere with policies, both in the areas of crime control and welfare, which tend to emphasise exclusion and the defence of boundaries (see Melossi 1980), to segregate problematic areas. Something of the type is portrayed in the film by John Carpenter *Escape From New York*: the ghettos as gigantic prisons, inside which reigns a do-it-yourself system of justice.

12   Another event is that of the privatisation of some American prisons, under the banner of cost saving and efficiency, experiments however, which for the most part are already failures.

13   The literature on this point is too vast and well known to be cited here. I refer rather to the interesting critical analysis and the methodological proposals which it arrives at, initiated by De Leonardis (1987), in which are identified, in contemporary social science, the beginnings of an overcoming of the actor–system dichotomy, thanks to an achievement of 'modesty' both in the conception of the actor and in that of the system.

14   Some of the stages of this relationship are examined in Foucault (1976) and in Galzigna (1984). The Italian positivist school, and, in this century, the school of 'social defence' attribute to 'science' a task primarily of the construction of law. Explicitly progressive and socialist substantivist currents give rise to periodic anti-formalist 'revolts' which, in the name of the primary necessity of combating inequality and injustice, draw on the repertoire and language of the social sciences. More generally, the tendency towards deformalisation in law as linked to the exigencies posed by the welfare state is discussed in Bobbio (1977).

15   Within the process itself however are intertwined the questions (and related discourses) of, as Geertz puts it (1988, chapter 8), 'what happened' and 'whether it was legal', or between the probatory and nominalistic dimensions of the sentencing process. In the chapters which follow the interconnection of these two dimensions of relation–conflict among 'experts' (psychiatrists, socio- logists, criminologists) and judges will be analysed from the standpoint of its outcome on the level of decisions and, indirectly, on the level of changes in professional standards and perceptions of one's own role by different categories of professionals.

16   The debate on the functions of punishment, in particular whether it should involve 'treatment' (intervention on the criminal to change him), arises, as has already been noted, with the modern criminal justice system. Retribution and treatment (however intended) cohabit from the beginning of the penitentiary institution, accompanying its changes and lending themselves to providing its justifications. For a history of penal policies in the welfare state, see Garland, 1985.

17   As will be seen further on, it is the same conception of 'treatment' that is changing, not least under the pressure of the transformation of need as a direct result of the enlargement of social citizenship. But there are also pressures more internal to the professions and bodies of knowledge concerning treatment which lead to the suspension or the radical reinterpretation of the objectives of

cure from the removal of symptoms or of the problems to the emphasis on the transformation of the problem itself, seeing the bearer of this problem as a protagonist of that transformation.

18 The history of welfare can be interpreted in relation to the requirements of ordering and disciplining the working classes, on the basis of the distinction, from the dawn of capitalist society, between the deserving and undeserving poor. See for example Foucault 1976; Piven and Cloward 1972; Rusche and Kirchheimer 1978; Chevalier, 1976.

19 The institution of Obligatory Medical Treatment for the mentally ill contained in the law on psychiatric reform (law 180 of 1978) is an example of the co-presence of these different rights and of the obligations which complementarity imposes on professionals (see Giannicheda 1986).

20 The paradoxes have been noted, in relation to this, of the so-called 'therapeutic contract' discussed by Dresser (1982): what happens when, knowingly suffering from recurrent psychotic crises during which I refuse treatment, I demand to be cured even if when I have need of it I don't want it? To which 'me' does the treatment refer? On the penal level similar questions are presented, where the lawfulness of the attribution of criminal responsibility is based on the presupposition of a continuity of personal identity: from the opposite standpoint one can read the process of criminal indictment as one of the construction of a personal identity responsible for the crime.

21 Analogous, on the other hand, is the interpretation given by functionalists and symbolic interactionists in terms of the stabilisation of shared expectations.

22 Fox Keller 1987, in an interrogation of the gendered (sexed) nature of science, proposes precisely this interpretation.

23 With the current legislative proposals (in the Italian Parliament) signed by the minister Russo Jervolino it will reacquire a status close to that of crime. On the other hand drug dependency presents a typically ambiguous face: on one hand it involves a choice, to make use of certain substances; on the other this use itself indicates an illness – of the 'mind' rather than the body – when dependence on the substance sets in. It is however this ambiguity which, if it is particularly visible in the case of drugs, is inherent in reality in many situations or conditions of daily life where choices and constraints intersect, so that what decides which of the two aspects predominates reveals itself as a political question in the broad sense, not delegable to any particular body of scientific knowledge.

24 An example is the Italian legislation concerning psychiatry, about which more will be said in a later chapter. More generally, questions of accountability are already raised within, and in relation to all, those institutions to which can be attributed functions of social control.

25 Although attempts in this sense have not been hitherto very encouraging (see Abel 1982).

26 On lines of principle, because the introduction of flexible penalties on one hand and the frequent vagueness and 'imprecision' of the legal formulations on the other, leave ample space for interpretation, arbitration, and therefore uncertainty as to the outcome.

27 It is also at the level of the relations between penal and social policy that the possibility exists of a minimal intervention justified in terms of 'efficiency', and, because efficient, in a position to defend the accused against unjust punishments.

RATHER RIDERS THAN HORSES?

1 I owe much, at least as far as the first part of this chapter is concerned, to the reflections, comments and suggestions of Stan Cohen. As one is accustomed to saying, errors and omissions are mine alone.

2 Here the discourse could get lengthy. Let us say that, beyond the evident differences, the crusade against child abuse alludes to themes which feminism and environmentalism have also used: a different relationship with, in fact a reinterpretation of the significance of, 'nature', a displacement of emphasis from a culture of acquisitiveness, performance and success to one of affection, emotion, closeness, etc.

3 See for example Becker 1987; Gusfield 1966, 1981; Pfohl 1973; Parton 1981; Walkowitz 1980.

4 This point is effectively discussed by De Leonardis 1988, p. 50.

5 The literature on identity is voluminous and differentiated. A substantial discussion and bibliography can be found in L. Balbo *et al.* 1985. See also Saraceno 1987a, for a critical reflection on the usefulness of this category.

6 On so-called 'everyday rights' including the right to the quality of life see Balbo 1987.

7 Is there more interpersonal violence today than, say, fifty years ago? Yes and no. No, if we limit ourselves to the statistics on violent crime. The violent settlement of interpersonal conflicts is a relatively rare event. The last three centuries of Western society indicate the progressive monopolisation by the state of the use of physical force. But the process of 'civilisation' simply shifts the attribution of violence to new acts and situations. The 'correction' of children becomes maltreatment and abuse. Dominant sexuality becomes violence and oppression. The disappearance of animal species becomes ecocide.

8 This is certainly not the only way in which they construct problems, neither are their activities reducible to the demands for criminalisation: but, when such demands are advanced, and for the period in which they are, they tend to attract into their orbit also other problems and activities which have feedback effects on the forms of organisation.

9 Ideally, of course. The extent, on the other hand, to which in reality being a poor, black and young male significantly affects the probability of being labelled as a criminal is something too well known to be dwelt on here.

10 An anything but simple option today, if for no other reason than because conflict about who is the victim most victimised (and therefore most merit worthy) is very open, and there are still many 'guilty' who participate.

11 Recently, the case of an underwater swimmer devoured by a shark in the sea off Tuscany has given rise to his being accused rather than to commiseration with the unfortunate victim: he was eaten because he frightened the poor shark, whose presence in our waters should be greeted with pleasure, even we Italians turn out to have some really wild animals . . .

12 Legitimation which can enter into conflict with the process of internal construction of a collective identity.

13 Which does not exclude desires, however legitimate, for punishment and even vengeance, which began to be expressed clearly in the years following the presentation, by the movement, of the proposed popular initiative on law reform. On this issue see the last chapter.

14 And, complementarily, to demand that the right to 'privacy' has priority over the protection of women. . . . See again, the last chapter for the polemic about mandatory prosecution and victim-initiated proceedings.

15 Something similar is happening on the thorny issue of the 'right to life'. Anti-abortionists and radical feminists, with apparently opposed motives, find themselves on the same platform (in the United States: but here in Italy we have already had an ambiguous taking of positions by environmentalists, not to speak of the presumed torments of conscience of many male socialists).

16 As far as the women's movement at least is concerned another reading of the ambivalence is possible. I reserve this discussion for the last chapter.

17 An example is that of the demand for compulsory care for drug addicts. The logic of the public agencies defines the drug takers as ill. The clients (or some of them) demand then a cure for this illness as a duty of the state, whether or not the patient wants it.

18 For the women's movement, which speaks for itself, interests and constructions of identity are much more strictly linked than in the other two cases; the environmentalists speak for all, the interests of which they declare themselves the bearers are widely diffused and the question of individual or group identity is more implicitly than directly in play. As far as the campaign against child abuse is concerned, here it betrays its affinity with many moral crusades, because it arises in the first instance within professional groups, psychologists, doctors, social workers, interested in extending the sphere of their own competence: for them, as a matter of principle, there is no conflict between 'internal' and 'external' identity.

19 The 'renaissance' (Bottoms 1977) of the category of social dangerousness is an indicator of this tendency. As I argued in the previous chapter, today the category of social dangerousness is used to identify 'populations at risk' (of committing crimes) within an ideology of punishment which legitimates its 'incapacitating' functions.

20 This phenomenon should however be examined in relation to the multiplication of groups and associations which arise in order to defend themselves from the intrusiveness, from the omnipotence, from the claimed irresponsibility of the large state and monopolistic providers of services, or from all those structures which, having an enormous influence on our lives, are difficult to get to assume responsibility towards us: consumers associations, councils for the rights of the sick etc. One of the fundamental characteristics of these associations is, again, the setting in motion of a process of assumption–attribution of responsibility.

21 The scapegoat 'theory', more or less subtended to those analyses of the campaigns of social alarm which interpret them as ways of diverting dissatisfactions and protests away from the centres of power, is not pertinent here. The symbolic nature of these processes of criminalisation lies in fact in the attempt to signify the presence of a conflict.

22 It is certainly a movement which during the 1980s acquired a great political influence. At the Federal level a President's Commission for the Victims of Crime (1984) was set up and a number of pieces of legislation enacted such as the Victim and Witness Protection Act (1982), Victims of Crime Act (1984) and the Justice Assistance Act (1984). In California a Victim's Bill of Rights was promulgated in 1982, following similar declarations in 28 other states. Forty-one states have programmes for victim compensation; but what counts more on the level of changes in the penal process is that many jurisdictions

admit some form of participation by the victim in judicial decisions concerning the guilty, for example the evaluation of the impact of the offence on the victim to establish the type and quantity of punishment. In California, the victims can also oppose the release on parole of the convicted. In general, victims demand preventive custody, speedy trials, the elimination of or the determination by victims themselves of plea-bargaining, reductions to the minimum of the power of cross examination of the victim by the defence, and participation in the decisions as to penalty (Henderson 1985).

23 Largely analogous are the associations of victims of the mafia and organised crime in general.

24 Indeed different, the consumer associations or councils for the rights of the sick, and similar. Not so much in terms of logic, which instead is analogous, as because they are true and properly established organisations.

THE QUESTION OF JUVENILE DEVIANCE

1 On juveniles see for example Cicourel 1968; Empey 1979; Krisberg, Austin 1978; Platt 1975; Schlossman 1977; on the mentally disabled see the discussion in the next chapter; on women, the bibliography in Pitch 1987.

2 For Italian research on juvenile justice see Faccioli, Pitch 1988; on the contemporary European context, Cain 1989; for a reflection and a biography on social control of women, see Pitch 1987.

3 The Italian sentencing system is a 'double track' system. One track is made up of 'punishments' (pene), the other of 'security measures'. Security measures may follow punishments, as in the case of being obliged to live in a certain place after the expiation of a prison sentence, or substitute punishments. To be referred to a psychiatric penitentiary hospital is a typical security measure given to adults released for reasons of insanity. Social dangerousness is the justification for security measures, while culpability is the justification for punishment. Punishment refers (in principle) to a judgement concerning the wilful commission of a criminal action, security measure refers to a judgement concerning the potential 'dangerousness', whether on social or psychological grounds, of an actor.

4 In this regard see Gatti, Bandini 1970; Senzani 1970; Ardigo' 1977; Bandini 1977; Balloni, Pellicciari, Sacchetti 1979; De Leo 1981; Censis 1982; Giasanti 1985; Ponti 1985; Giasanti, Calabretta 1987.

5 Periodically, media reports and investigations are made on juvenile delinquency in those Southern areas where organised crime is more flourishing. Whether or not all, or most, of the crimes committed by youth in those areas (Palermo, Naples) are connected to or directed by organised criminal groups, they are different from those supposedly characterising the delinquency of juvenile gangs. First of all, there are rarely gangs. Youths are usually not autonomously organised, and they do not engage in fights against each other. Their crimes are property crimes, often related to illegal activities engaged in by the adults of the area. Media and public opinion concern is mainly directed to this connection, and police and judges often point out the use that adults make of children in criminal activities, as children under 14 are not punishable. Another problem discussed is that of gypsy children, both girls and boys. Gypsy children are often used as beggars and bag-snatchers, and of course they are very visible and an easy object of attention on the part of the police (see Faccioli, Pitch 1988). As immigration from North Africa, Eastern Europe and

other countries increases, there is a steady increase in the rate of adult incarceration of people from these countries. It is to be expected that such an increase will happen for juveniles too, and that soon, when in Italy as well there will be recognisable 'ethnic minorities', the whole question will take on different characteristics.

6 The new code of juvenile criminal procedure, on which I will make some remarks further on, insists in fact on the importance of the 're-educative' goals of juvenile justice.

7 The prevalence of verdicts of immaturity in Southern Italy by comparison with Northern Italy gives rise to the thought that they are used both to highlight the consequences of family and social structures which are as precarious as they are widespread, and to stimulate intervention by public social services.

8 The nearest equivalent in English legal terminology to the concept of 'incapacity of understanding and intention' would be 'unfit to plead'. However they are not the same concept. The Italian notion of incapacity refers to the issue of free will from a juridical and philosophical point of view rather than the capacity of the individual to actually stand trial.

9 See Cappuccio, Curti Gialdino 1985; Dosi 1985; Mazzei 1984; Ponti 1985; Santarsiero 1985; Sergio 1982; Spagnoletti 1985.

10 Though, naturally, fulfilling them in practice: something very similar happens for the mental health services in relation to psychiatric patients who have problems with the law. I will discuss this at greater length in the next chapter.

11 In a piece of research on a year's activity by the juvenile public prosecutor of Rome, a good percentage of juveniles, and especially girls, were charged with driving without a licence (Faccioli, Pitch 1988).

12 It is evident from the research mentioned in note 11, that gypsies are treated more severely by juvenile judges for equivalent crimes, than Italian youth (see also Cipollini, Faccioli and Pitch 1989). It is a question here, in my opinion, of the result of two interlinked phenomena: of an increasingly frequent attribution of dangerousness to gypsies as criminal justice becomes the unique and necessary arrival point for a problem which other agencies have not wanted to or not known how to handle, and at the same time of a process of redefinition, on the part of judges, of their proper role in terms of a penal orientation such as to both confirm the symbolic function of punishment and to legitimate their own function.

13 A good example of these are, again, gypsies.

CRIMINAL RESPONSIBILITY AND MENTAL ILLNESS

1 The research, conducted together with O. De Leonardis, G. Gallio, and D. Mauri, refers to the sub-project 'illnesses of the nervous system' of the National Council of Research. To this project was assigned objective No. 30 'census of the handicapped by serious psychiatric illness' which was identified as the analysis of that area of urban social handicap characterised by the co-presence of psychic suffering and socially disruptive behaviour, and is defined and delimited by relations and competences which reciprocate between psychiatry and criminal justice. In this chapter I refer in particular to that part of the research which had as its object the relations between judges, forensic psychiatric experts and mental health services at Milan through interviews by means of questionnaires, depth discussions and content analyses of two samples of psychiatric reports in criminal proceedings during the years 1971–2

and 1981–2. Much of what I will say is therefore the result of common labour, which has among other things as its first result the volume by De Leonardis *et al.* 1988 *Curare e Punire*, Milan, Unicopli 1988 and numerous articles by individual members of the research group, to which I will frequently refer.

2   Law 180, 1978 is a law that 'civilises' psychiatry, not in the sense that it makes it up to date, but in the sense that it privileges its therapeutic and medical vocation, and cuts its ties with custody and control. Such ties were embodied by the asylum, the psychiatric hospital – an institution geared to take in charge those problems (and that population) that fell outside the boundaries set by medicine and criminal justice. Mental illness, poverty, social disturbance, marginality, different types of body handicaps and much else were all contained by the asylum and taken in charge by psychiatry. The asylum was the embodiment of the link established between cure and custody, legitimated by that other link, that between mental illness and social dangerousness. Asylum psychiatry constructed itself upon these links. Law 180 dissolves them. Already in the early 1970s the previous law regulating psychiatry, which dated back to 1904, was partly changed by abolishing forced confinement in an asylum. Law 180 provides for the gradual closing down of all types of custodial and long-term residential institutions for the mentally ill and for treatment to be obtained through community mental health services, which should substitute entirely for asylums. It establishes the principle that to be treated is a right, and therefore that nobody can be treated, for whatever reason, against her consent, and that therefore the links between mental illness and social dangerousness, cure and custody, are rescinded. Persons suffering with some kind of mental disturbance are fully citizens, whose rights must be respected.

3   Translator's note: see note 8 to chapter 'The question of juvenile deviance'.

4   This chapter does not deal with the question of guilt, or the subjective aspects of the offence from the standpoint of penal science, a question which is today the focus of attention by jurists in various countries and in which the theme of criminal responsibility is central. For a discussion see in particular: Fiandaca 1987; Silbernagl 1987. I will limit myself here to that aspect of criminal responsibility which is concerned with liability and I will obviously treat it as a sociologist rather than as a jurist. (See Bertolino 1988; Pulitanò 1988.)

5   As I already explained in the preceding chapter, the Italian system of punishment is a two-track system. 'Punishments' are given on the basis of the commission of actions defined as crimes, 'security measures' are given on the basis of a judgement of 'social dangerousness' regarding certain characteristics of the individual who has committed illegal actions. If a court finds that a crime has been committed by somebody who was 'incapable of understanding and wanting' at the time the crime was committed, it must acquit him. It must then decide whether that individual is 'socially dangerous'. If it so decides, then it must apply a 'security measure', usually confinement to a penal psychiatric hospital, for a period specified in its minimum but not in its maximum. Up until a Constitutional Court sentence in 1982, 'social dangerousness' was 'presumed', i.e. automatically associated with an acquittal on the basis of insanity. Since 1982, 'social dangerousness' must be 'proven' in each case.

6   The critical analysis of the effects of psychiatrisation of the community as the result of de-institutionalisation is analogous to that which many sociologists of social control have conducted on the effects of decarceration, decriminalisation, community control etc. See Castel *et al.* 1979; Cohen 1979; Scull 1977.

7 See for example Canepa 1985; Bandini 1988; Gatti 1988; Bandini, Gatti 1985; Debuyst 1981; Harding 1980; Pfohl 1978; Ponti 1985.

8 I remember, as far as Italy is concerned, among the many meetings devoted to these arguments, the seminar on incapacity to comprehend and will which took place at Gragnano in 1984, and the 5th national seminar for Italian criminologists, entirely on this theme, held at Syracuse in 1986. In addition the seventh criminological colloquium of the Council of Europe *'Etudes sur la responsabilité penale et le traitement psychiatrique des delinquants malades mentaux'*, Strasbourg, November 1985.

9 The research has additionally concerned itself with the lower courts (equivalent to English magistrates courts, though presided over by normal professional judges identical to those of the higher courts (see De Leonardis 1988b; Gandus 1988). These are particularly significant because these are nowadays the principal landing place and clearing house, within the criminal justice system, for offences relating to public nuisance and breach of the peace, and of the psychiatrically handicapped. Another observation point has been the hospital of San Vittore (see Mauri, Pitch 1990). Also, the research at Trieste is continuing.

10 An apparent paradox is to be noted here, and has been discussed by Philippe Robert, namely that the scientific delegitimation of the notion of social dangerousness has been accompanied by an increase in its use. It is in fact really its disconnection from naturalistic presuppositions which facilitates a more generalised, diffuse and increasingly discretionary deployment, subordinated to the requirements of 'social defence'.

11 Since I first wrote this passage much has, apparently, changed. I refer to the dominant role of the Italian judiciary in the collapse of the political establishment which ruled Italy since 1948. The result has been simultaneously an enhanced independence of the judiciary from the political system and of the political impact of the judiciary itself. Indeed, in times of manifest weakness of official political actors and institutions, the judiciary and the criminal justice system appear to invade the scene, and take over the missing functions. This occurred during the terrorism emergency of the 1970s. It has happened even more strongly in the past two years. Legal changes have also taken place. The new code of criminal procedure, which should have introduced an adversarial system in Italy, in place of the traditional inquisitorial one, has already been amended at various points with the effect of mitigating precisely its adversarial orientation. A new law (1990) re-criminalising drug use was amended by referendum (1993), making drug use, while an offence, yet again non-punishable. A change in the psychiatric reform law, reintroducing residential compulsory care, was discussed in Parliament, though it has not yet been approved. Everything seems to be in flux today in Italy, not only at the institutional level, but even more at the cultural one. Yet, though so much has changed, and it is difficult to interpret the direction and extension of this change, I think that the main elements sustaining my interpretation of the relationships between the criminal justice and welfare systems stand unaltered.

12 This characteristic results both from the analysis of expert psychiatric judgements of the years 1981–2 as compared to those of 1971–2, and from the responses of the judges of the Milan court to our questionnaire, in relation to the requests for expert psychiatric opinions during 1986. It was confirmed by the judges and by the psychiatric experts that we interviewed.

13 In recent years, two proposals for legislation (bill 177 of 1983 and 3260 of 1985) in delineating the mode of abolition of asylums for the criminally insane, propose the abolition of non-liability due to mental illness and, in fact, an equal treatment as regards punishment for both the mentally ill and those of sound mind. The cornerstone of the proposal, much discussed, is the idea of the restoration to the mentally ill of responsibility for their own actions, as a process which is both in itself therapeutic as well as respecting the civil rights of the mentally ill themselves.

14 The expert judgements relating to the years 1971 and 1972 were 21, those relating to 1981 and 1982 were 32. The latter refer predominantly to young adult males (27), mainly single residents in the Milan region, with low educational achievement, unemployed or intermittently employed. Of these, 19 had a psychiatric history previous to the judgement which took the form of brief repetitive confinements in civil psychiatric hospitals. Fourteen were known to the courts, arising from numerous reported offences and several arrests, but without prolonged detention. The repertoire of offences for which they were indicted is rather large: four homicides and six attempted murders, four indictments of cruelty, and three of threatening behaviour, six robberies and an assortment of other offences, obscene behaviours, resisting public officials. (Translator's note: these are of course offence categories from the Italian criminal code and not necessarily directly translatable into English offences.) As far as victims were concerned, they were generally family members, friends, neighbours, acquaintances, in addition to public officials. The cases of the previous decade refer to younger males, with a higher level of education, in employment which, even if low paid, was better and more stable than that revealed ten years later. The range of offences was also smaller and less serious: a prevalence of violence and cruelty, and some thefts. The requests for expert judgement were here more directly linked to the awareness of a preceding psychiatric history. In 1981–2 the experts diagnosed 15 cases of partial mental defect and seven cases of total mental incapacity. Eight were diagnosed as in full capacity, while there were four diagnoses of full capacity at the time of the assessment linked to partial defect at the time of the offence. There were many more diagnoses of total mental incapacity in the two years 1971–2.

15 These hypotheses emerged from our meetings with judges and forensic psychiatrists.

16 Particular cases are on the one hand the so-called (and deplored) improper use of psychiatric reports in relation to members of organised crime (for a commentary on the entire debate, in forensic psychiatry, on the simulation of illness and the ways of identifying it see Fornari 1986). On the other hand the lower courts, which since 1986 are in charge of a larger quota of crimes than before, among which are most offences relating to general public disturbance, of petty crime and small neighbourhood and family conflicts, receive the largest number of cases at the boundaries of psychiatry and law (vagabonds, tramps, addicts, ex-psychiatric patients, etc.). Many of the testimonies we gathered among the judges of the Milanese lower court indicated a general reluctance to have recourse to psychiatric expertise in the conviction that such intervention can only aggravate the position of the accused, being the prelude to a confinement in a penal psychiatric hospital seen as obligatory in the case of a judgement of dangerousness (see Gandus 1988; De Leonardis 1988b). Today it is the judges, under the new accelerated trial system, who play the principal role in

deciding on 'grey' situations and who increasingly, in a game of delegation of responsibilities, apply the decisions concerning the destiny of those whom the services cannot or will not follow up, whom the police do not know what to do with, or families or neighbours cannot put up with.

17 In our research in the Milan courts we sought both by means of interviews and the administration of questionnaires to evaluate how far the reform of psychiatry and more generally the changes in psychiatric culture were understood and evaluated by criminal court judges and how far and in what ways it had affected their decisions in relation to liability and social dangerousness and their relations with forensic psychiatric experts; and whether such changes had led to the establishment of relations with community psychiatric centres and if and how they have modified the judges' perception of penal psychiatric hospitals.

18 Of the questionnaires sent by us directly, and solicited personally, only 20 were completed. These consisted of 10 sub-prosecutors and investigating judges, six magistrates and four appeal judges. The questionnaire was divided into two parts. The first attempted to establish the number of expert reports requested during 1986, the motives for which they had been requested, the criteria for the choice of expert, the level of rapport with the experts themselves, the outcome of the cases to which the advice referred. The second part was aimed at registering the attitude and opinion of the judge with respect to the relation between mental illness, incapacity and social dangerousness, to the penal psychiatric hospital, to the prospect of an introduction of a criminological expertise – linked neither to mental illness, nor to establishing only mental capacity and dangerousness, but aimed at describing the personality and history of the defendant and, in principle, applicable to all defendants.

19 By integrated criminal science is meant that model of the science of criminal law, still dominant in Italy, which is based on the integration of juridical dogmatics with the social sciences existing in Italy between the turn of the century and the 1930s: criminology and psychiatry of a positivist imprint (see Baratta 1979).

20 We know this, from, among other sources, the meetings and interviews with judges.

21 It is different, for example, to base one's intervention on the basis of a model oriented to cure, understood as the disappearance of all symptoms, or on one directed towards cure, understood as an instrument for putting 'patients' in a position to live to the best of their possibilities.

22 These things are often done also by the agencies which base themselves on the first model, only that they are seen as extraneous to their proper competences and obligations and as therefore distorting the meaning of their proper mandate.

23 Partly analogous problems are encountered nevertheless in the handling and care of any infectious illness, such as venereal disease and today HIV/AIDS.

24 Law 180 allows for a Compulsory Medical Treatment Order for a period of no more than fifteen days to be administered in *ad hoc* psychiatric sections of normal hospitals in exceptional cases. The city mayor's official assent is necessary for any such Order. Doctors administering treatment under such an Order should – according to the law – actively seek the patient's consent to treatment.

25 This is what for example, has been demanded by some of the practitioners in Perugia, after the case began.

FROM OPPRESSION TO VICTIMISATION

1   Prior to the approval of this law, in 1958, prostitution was legal if, and only if, exercised in State licensed brothels. Prostitutes were given a card (*tessera*) stating their status, and were obliged to subject themselves to periodical health checks. When found ill, they were confined in hospitals for venereal diseases (*sifilicomi*). Under this system, prostitutes circulated from one brothel to another (the usual period of stay was fifteen days), and paid the owners for their food and lodgings, and for whatever else they needed to survive, which meant that very few of them succeeded in laying aside enough money to either leave the trade or set up their own brothels. The windows of brothels had to be permanently shut, and that is why they were commonly called *case chiuse*, closed houses. Different categories of brothels existed, each with its fixed tariff. Hours of work were long and rules very rigid. Prostitutes were virtual recluses in these houses. As prostitution was illegal outside licensed brothels (which, of course, regularly paid taxes), the so-called morals police (*polizia del buoncostume*) had among its tasks precisely that of looking for prostitutes on the street and arresting them, whereby they would be given a card and be obliged to work in brothels. Obviously, police persecution and blackmail were common, and many cases are documented of 'innocent' women having been harassed, blackmailed, arrested, and given cards (which amounted to indelible stigmatisation) by the police.

2   Henceforth, I shall use the term abolitionists to indicate those political forces which were in favour of the abolition of the State regulation of prostitution, i.e. of the existing system; I shall use the term regulationists to indicate those political forces who were in favour of the maintenance of the existing regulatory regime.

3   The references to the debates and draft legislation are as follows: Senato, I legislatura, Documentazione – Disegni di legge, n.63-A, p. 12. The relevant Parliamentary documents examined are: Senato, I legislatura: Documentazioni – Disegni di legge – relazioni, 1948, n.63 e 63-A. Discussioni: 12-10-1949, pp. 10801–10824; 28-9-1949, pp. 10379–10397; 5-3-1952, pp. 31375–31401; 24-3-1950, pp. 14813–14918. Senato, II legislatura: Documentazioni-Disegni di legge – Relazioni, 1953, n.28. Discussioni: 21-1-1955, pp. 305–333. Camera, I legislatura: Documentazioni – Disegni di legge – Relazioni, 1952, n.2602-A. Camera, II legislatura: Documentazioni – Disegni di legge – Relazioni, 1956, n.1439-A. Discussioni: 28-1-1958, pp. 39345–39367; 29-1-1958, pp. 39419–39420.

4   Analogous 'misunderstandings' have occurred more recently in relation to law 194 on abortion, which was criticised for not having among its objectives the disappearance of abortion. This is a recurrent misunderstanding. Similarly, in the interests of a speedy approval of the law on sexual violence, claims were made as to a presumed efficacy in containing or reducing the phenomenon. Likewise various changes and about turns concerning legislation on drug use were justified in the name of a greater efficacy in reducing the phenomenon: the omnipotence of the law! Or rather, on one hand opportunism, on the other an incapacity to distinguish between the objective of eliminating the consequences of criminalisation and that of eliminating the phenomenon itself as the aim of these laws.

5   This seems to be the destiny of those campaigns and laws, initially driven by civic values (the termination of a particular regime degrading for prostitutes,

the protection of sexual freedom) which intervene in the traditional relations between the sexes. Even the new bill on sexual violence speaks increasingly, after ten years of struggle, the language of the disciplining of sexuality, of the intervention of authority to limit what is perceived as danger, rather than that of the protection of rights to liberty, even in this sphere. How else is legislation which provides for the punishment of those who intentionally let juveniles see sexual acts to be understood?

6 See for example McNickle 1977; Rafter 1985; Walkowitz 1987.
7 The resemblance to the struggles against regulation of the second half of the nineteenth century is truly impressive. See Gibson 1987.

FROM VICTIMISATION TO AUTONOMY

1 For some recent data on Italy see Canepa, Lagazzi 1988; Ventimiglia 1987.
2 For an analagous position, inasmuch as it is based on an attempt to 'ground' the concept of social injury see Feltsiner, Abel, Sarat 1980–81.
3 The sociological and psychological literature on rape born in the wake of the women's movment is by now enormous. Some indicative contributions are: Brownmiller 1975; McKinnon 1987; Schwendinger, Schwendinger 1983; for Italy, the excellent contribution by Ventimiglia 1987.
4 The almost contemporaneous (1988) stories of the reaction of an American and of a Sicilian town to sexual violence suffered by two girls are, from this point of view, unedifying. In the case of both Tawana in the United States and Pina in Sicily the greater part of their co-citizens lined up against them, accusing the girls of lying and national public opinion of racism.
5 See however Davis, Anderson 1983, where the structures of self-help, even those which receive official recognition and finance are analysed as mechanisms for the diffusion of 'social control' but of a control 'alternative' to that of the institutions: decentralised, informal, reciprocal, participatory.
6 I am speaking here about heterosexuality because lesbianism has been, not by chance, rather more talked about and reflected upon by women, as a sexual orientation in itself subversive of dominant sexuality. Nevertheless the question of violence in sexuality, understood as possibility and pleasure from relations of domination and submission, concerns and has been discussed with regard to relations between women as well as those between men and women. (e.g. Rubin 1981). As far as alternatives to dominant heterosexuality are concerned, there circulate not so much thought out reflections as prescriptions and censures of type: 'women want a sexuality which is sweet, tender, egalitarian, non-aggressive'.
7 The contents of the proposals for the popular initiative for law reform were: the shifting of the crimes of sexual violence from Title XI of the Penal Code (crimes against morality) to Title XII (crimes against the person); the unification into a single crime of the crime of carnal violence and acts of violent lust (meaning: rape involving actual penetration in the vagina, on the one hand, and all other types of rape, on the other); mandatory prosecution; the admission as plaintiffs of 'movements and associations for the liberation of women'.
8 I have recounted this history in Pitch 1983a. To summarise briefly: the idea of a popular initiative for law reform was born following the experience of a Centre run by the Movement for Women's Liberation (MLD) after a notorious brutal group rape in 1975. In the September of 1978 there took place in Rome

an international conference of women on rape in which it was decided to conduct a survey. The results were 'disturbing': 92.2 per cent of the women who responded had 'suffered physical, sexual or emotional violence' (see Lagostena Bassi 1979). From this survey the MLD drew its arguments which formed the basis of the proposal for legal reform which was presented in April 1979. In the autumn the Roman Feminist Movement (MFR), the UDI and the MLD formed a joint committee to promote the reform after the election of a new parliament. The political parties also presented their proposals. The first was the PCI, in 1977 (it is useful perhaps to remember that, in this first initiative, victim-initiated proceedings were retained). Between 1979 and 1980 all the other parties followed suit.

9 See for example, many of the interventions at the conference 'Against Sexual Violence, Women and the Law', held at Milan on 27 and 28 October 1979 (duplicated report).

10 On the internal contradictions of the popular initiative for legal reform and successive parliamentary initiatives, especially regarding the relationships universality–specificity, autonomy–protection, see Pitch 1983a, 1984, 1985.

11 I refer to seduction with promise of marriage and infanticide for reasons of honour.

12 Naturally, this contradiction, implicit in each struggle for emancipation, is inevitable. But if one were conscious of it, and in fact it was acted out in the preceding struggles – abortion for example – in this case it was neither acted out nor recognised. (See Pitch 1983a.)

13 The polemic appears, besides in the various documents edited by the collectives, such as the resolutions of the Milan conference, in the pages of the daily newspaper *Il Manifesto* during the autumn and winter of 1979–80, in the journal *Noi Donne* and in the newspaper *Lotta Continua* of the same period. See also 'Un dibattito sulla proposta del movimento delle donne', (a debate on the women's movement proposal) in *Politica del Diritto*, XI, 3, 1980.

14 The law approved by the Senate in the June of 1988 additionally reintroduced presumed violence in the case of minors. In the Chamber of Deputies, the justice commission succeeded again in reintroducing mandatory prosecution in all cases and in lowering the age threshold in which sexual relations are admitted to take place between minors.

15 Curiously, only a couple of years after this was written, a prime time Italian TV movie shown on public TV told a story which developed this very theme. During a rape trial, after the lawyers of the accused have used all the usual derogatory repertoire against the victim, the mother of the accused rises to denounce him and stand by the victim.

16 In different terms, this dichotomy has been affirmed by Heidensohn 1986, when she demands a different justice for women. See the answer by Daly, 1989; also, Klein 1988, 1991. Klein suggests that, in approaching the question of criminal justice from the point of view of women, we take into account at the same time women authors of crime and women victims of crime. I consider this approach very fruitful, in that it allows one to pose the issue of responsibility, and, consequently, of justice, in such a way as to overcome the dichotomy between relational and abstract responsibility and 'rehabilitation' and 'punishment'. I developed this argument more in Pitch 1992.

17 A discussion on equality in law as, simultaneously, presupposition and prescription, rule and decision, can be found in Resta 1985. The tension

established between the two aspects is not only what signifies co-presence of and conflict between formal equality and (policies aimed at) substantive equality: it can be usefully explored in relation to a project for gendered law.

A POLITICS OF SOVEREIGNTY

1 The current debate on redistributive justice and welfare policies is too vast to be noted here. Martha Minow's excellent book on the paradoxes of equality policies and rights-oriented approaches, and her suggestion of a social relational approach (Minow 1990) and Amartya Sen's suggestion of policies based on a right to fundamental capabilities (Sen 1985) appear to me to be well within what I have called a politics of sovereignty. De Leonardis' (1990) contributions on these questions are also very illuminating.

Bibliography

AA.VV. (1977) 'Ordine e democrazia nella crisi: un dibattito interno alla sinistra', *La questione criminale*, III, 2.

AA.VV. (1979) 'Terrorismo e stato della crisi', *La questione criminale*, V, 1.

AA.VV. (1982) *Riposte giudiziarie alla criminalità minorile*, Unicopli, Milan.

AA.VV. (1986–7) 'A "Social Issue" in American Politics: Reflections on Kristin Luker's *Abortion and the Politics of Motherhood*', *Politics and Society*, XV, 2, 189–234.

Abel, R. (1979) 'Delegalization: a Critical Review of its Ideology and Social Consequences', in E. Blankenburg *et al.* (eds), *Alternative Rechtsformen und Alternative zum Recht. Jahrbuch für Recchssoziologie*, band 6, Westdeutscher Verlag, Opladen.

Abel, R. (1982) 'The Contradictions of Informal Justice', in R.L. Abel (ed.), *The Politics of Informal Justice*, Academic Press, New York.

Abel, R.L. (1982a) 'Torts', in D. Kairys (ed.), *The Politics of Law*, Pantheon, New York.

Allen, H. (1988) 'One Law for All Reasonable Persons?', *The International Journal of the Sociology of Law*, XVI, 4, 419–432.

American Friends Service Committee Working Party (1971), *Struggle for Justice. A Report on Crime and Punishment in America*, Hill and Wang, New York.

Amir, M. (1971) *Patterns of Forcible Rape*, Chicago University Press, Chicago.

Ardigò, A. (1977) (ed.), *Giustizia minorile e famiglia*, Patron, Bologna.

Arendt, H. (1989) *Vita Activa*, Bologna, Il Mulino.

Ariès, P. (1974) *Padri e figli nell'Europa medievale e moderna*, Laterza, Bari.

Bailey, R., Brake, M. (1975) *Radical Social Work*, Edward Arnold, London.

Balbo, L. (1987) (ed.), *Time to care*, Franco Angeli, Milan.

Balbo, L. *et al.* (1985) *Complessità sociale e identità*, Franco Angeli, Milan.

Balloni, A., Pellicciari, G., Sacchetti, L. (1979) *Devianza e giustizia minorile*, Franco Angeli, Milan.

Bandini, T. (1977) 'Considerazioni sulle attuali tendenze della delinquenza giovanile', *Rassegna di Criminologia*, VIII, 1/2, 25–34.

Bandini, T. (1988) 'Il contributo del clinico al dibattito sulla psichiatria e sugli ospedali psichiatrici giudiziari', in O. De Leonardis, G. Gallio, D. Mauri, T. Pitch (eds), *Curare e punire*, Unicopli, Milan.

Bandini, T., Gatti, U. (1982) 'Perizia psichiatrica e perizia criminologica: riflessioni sul ruolo del perito nell'ambito del processo penale', *Rivista italiania di medicina legale*, 13, 321–330.

Bandini, T., Gatti, U. (1985) 'Psichiatria e giustizia. Riflessioni critiche sull'imputabilità del malato di mente', *Dei delitti e delle pene*, III, 2, 351.

Bandini, T., Gatti, U. (1987) *Delinquenza giovanile*, Giuffré, Milan.

Baratta, A. (1979) 'Criminologia e dogmatica penale. Passato e futuro del modello integrato di scienza penalistica', *La questione criminale*, V, 2, 147–183.

Baratta, A. (1982) *Criminologia critica e critica del diritto penale*, Il Mulino, Bologna.

Barratta, A. (1985) 'Principi del diritto penale minimo. Per una teoria dei diritti umani come oggetti e limiti della legge', *Dei delitti e delle pene*, III, 3, 443–473.

Barratta, A., Silbernagl, M. (1983) 'La legislazione dell'emergenza e la cultura giuridica garantista nel processo penale', *Dei delitti e delle pene*, I, 3, 543–580.

Barsotti, A., Calcagno, G., Losana, C., Vercellone, P. (1976) 'Sull'imputabilità dei minori tra i 14 e i 18 anni', *Esperienze di rieducazione*, XXVII, 2–3, 18–44.

Becker, H. (1987) *Outsiders*, Edizioni Gruppo Abele, Turin.

Bergonzini, L., Pavarini, M., (1985) (eds), *Potere giudiziario, enti locali e giustizia minorale*, Il Mulino, Bologna.

Berlin, I. (1969) *Four Essays on Liberty*, Oxford, Oxford University Press.

Bertolino, M. (1988) 'La questione attuale dell'imputabilità penale', in O. De Leonardis, G. Gallio, D. Mauri, T. Pitch (eds), *Curare e punire*, Unicopli, Milan.

Betti, M., Pavarini, M. (1984) 'La tutela sociale della/dalla follia. Note teoriche sulla scienza psichiatrica di fronte alle nuove strategie di controllo sociale', *Dei delitti e delle pene*, II, 1, 161–183.

Bienen, L. (1983) 'Rape Reform Legislation in the United States', *Victimology*, 8, 139–151.

Bobbio, N. (1977) *Dalla struttura alla funzione*, Comunità, Milan.

Bocchetti, A. (1984) 'Perché ho paura degli uomini', *Il Manifesto*, 3 November.

Boccia, M.L. (1989) 'L'eguaglianza impermeabile. Il corpo femminile ridisegna l'orizzonte dei diritti eguali', *il Bimestrale*, 1, 81–86.

Boccia, M.L. (1989) '"Singolaritá", "pluralitá" e genere nee femminismo', *Reti*, 3–4.

Boccia, M.L., Peretti, I. (1988) (eds), *Il genere della rappresentanza*, Supplemento al n. 1 di *Democrazia e diritto*, Editori Riuniti, Rome.

Bono, P., Kemp, S. (1990) *Italian Feminist Thought*, London, Basil Blackwell.

Bono, P., Kemp, S. (1992) *The Lonely Mirror*, London, Routledge.

Bottoms, A. (1977) 'Reflections on the Renaissance of Dangerousness', *Howard Journal of Penology and Crime Prevention*, 16, 2, 70–96.

Bottoms, A. (1983) 'Neglected Features of Contemporary Penal Systems', in D. Garland, P. Young (eds), *The Power to Punish*, Heinemann, London.

Boudon, R. (1980) *Effetti perversi dell'azione sociale*, Feltrinelli, Milan.

Box-Grainger, J. (1986) 'Sentencing Rapists', in R. Matthews, J. Young, *Confronting Crime*, Sage, London.

Bredemeier, H.C. (1962) 'The Law as an Integrative Mechanism', in W. Evan (ed.), *Law and Sociology*, The Free Press of Glencoe, New York.

Bricola, F. (1982) 'Il pentimento del terrorista, il perdono all'evasore e i silenzi della legge n. 646 del 1982', *Politica del diritto* 4, 493–498.

Brownmiller, S. (1975) *Against Our Will. Men, Women and Rape*, Simon and Schuster, New York.

Buttafuoco, A. (1984) *Le mariuccine. Storia di un'istituzione laica*, Franco Angeli, Milan.

Cain, M. (1985) 'Beyond Informal Justice', *Contemporary Crises*, 9, 4, 335–373.

Cain, M. (1989) (ed.), *Growing Up Good*, Sage, London.

Campari, M.G., Cigarini, L. (1989) 'Fonte e principi di un nuovo diritto', in Libreria delle donne di Milano (ed.), *Un filo di felicità, Sottosopra*, January.

Canepa, G. (1985) 'Aspetti problematici ed esigenze di riforma della perizia psichiatrica', Relazione al Convegno su *L'istituzione psichiatrica giudiziaria nel servizio sanitario nazionale*, Castiglione delle Stiviere, 25–28 March.

Canepa, G., Lagazzi, M. (1988) (eds), *I delitti sessuali*, Cedam, Padova.

Canosa, R., Sacco, D., Sacco, M.P. (1987) 'Perizia psichiatrica e gioco delle parti', in M.G. Giannichedda, F. Ongaro Basaglia (eds), *Psichiatria, tossico-dipendenze, perizia*, Franco Angeli, Milan.

Cappuccio, N., Curti Gialdino, F. (1985) 'L'immaturità come variabile territoriale?', *Esperienze di giustizia minorile*, XXXII, 1, 107–111.

Caringella-MacDonald, S. (1988) 'Marxist and Feminist Interpretations on the Aftermath of Rape Reform', *Contemporary Crises*, XII, 2, 125–143.

Cassano, F. (1971) *Autocritica della sociologia contemporanea*, De Donato, Bari.

Castel, F., Castel, R., Lovell, A. (1979) *La société psychiatrique avancée*, Grasset, Paris.

Cavarero, A. (1988) 'L'ordine dell'uno non è l'ordine del due', in M.L. Boccia, I. Peretti (eds), *Il genere della rappresentanza*, Editori Runiti, Rome.

Cavarero, A. (1988a) 'Leggendo Irigaray', *Fluttuaria*, 5, 17–18.

Cavarero, A. (1992) 'Hannah Arendt: la libertà come bene comune', *Democrazia e diritto*, n. 5–6.

Censis (1982) *Indagine nazionale sull'andamento e sulle attuali tendenze della devianza minorile*, Rome.

Chapman, D. (1971) *Lo stereotipo del criminale*, Einaudi, Turin.

Chevalier, L. (1976) *Classi lavoratrici e classi pericolose*, Laterza, Bari.

Christie, N. (1985) *Abolire le pene? Il paradosso del sistema penale*, Edizioni Gruppo Abele, Turin.

Cicourel, A.V. (1968) *The Social Organization of Juvenile Justice*, John Wiley, New York.

Cipollini, R., Faccioli, F., Pitch, T. (1989) 'Gipsy Girls in an Italian Juvenile Court', in M. Cain (ed.) *Growing Up Good*, Sage, London.

Cohen, A. (1955) *Ragazzi delinquenti*, Feltrinelli, Milan.

Cohen, S. (1979) 'The Punitive City: Notes on the Dispersal of Social Control', *Contemporary Crises*, III, 4, 339–363.

Cohen, S. (1983) 'Social Control Talk. Telling Stories about Correctional Change', in D. Garland, P. Young (eds), *The Power to Punish*, Heinemann, London.

Cohen, S. (1985) *Visions of Social Control*, Polity Press, Cambridge.

Cohen, S. (1988) 'Taking Decentralization Seriously', 213–234, in S. Cohen, *Against Criminology*, Transaction, Inc., New Brunswick.

Cohen, S. (1988a) *Against Criminology*, Transaction, Inc., New Brunswick.

Cohen, S. (1988b) 'The Object of Criminology', in S. Cohen, *Against Criminology*, Transaction, Inc., New Brunswick.

Cohen, S., Scull, A. (eds) (1983) *Social Control and the State*, Martin Robertson, Oxford.

Cuomo, M.P., La Greca, G., Viggiani, L. (1982) (eds), *Giudici, psicologi e delinquenza giovanile*, Giuffré, Milan.

Daga, L. (1985) 'Ospedali psichiatrici giudiziari, sistema penale e sistema penitenziario', *Rassegna penitenziaria e criminologica*, 1/3, 1–52.

Daly, K. (1989) 'Criminal Justice Ideologies and Practices in Different Voices:

Some Feminist Questions about Justice', *The International Journal of the Sociology of Law*, n.1.

Daly, M. (1978) *Gyn/Ecology, The Metaethics of Radical Feminism*, Beacon Press, Boston.

Davis, M. (1983) 'How to Make Punishment Fit the Crime', *Ethics*, 93, 726–752.

Davis, N.J., Anderson, B. (1983) *Social Change. The Production of Deviance in the Modern State*, Irvington, New York.

De Giorgi, R. (1984) *Azione e imputazione*, Milella, Bari.

De Leo, G. (1981) *La giustizia dei minori*, Einaudi, Turin.

De Leo, G. (1985) 'Per una definizione della responsabilità minorile', *Esperienze di giustizia minorile*, XXXII, 1, 115–149.

De Leo, G., Cuomo, M.P. (1983) *La delinquenza minorile come rappresentazione sociale*, Marsilio, Venice.

De Leonardis, O. (1987) 'Percorsi cognitivi tra attore sociale e sistema', relazione presentata al seminario della sezione *Riproduzione sociale, vita quotidiana e soggetti collettivi* dell'Associazione Italiana di Sociologia, 10 October, Bologna.

De Leonardis, O. (1988) 'Statuto e figure della pericolosità sociale tra psichiatria riformata e giustizia penale', in O. De Leonardis, G. Gallio, D. Mauri, T. Pitch, *Curare e punire*, Unicopli, Milan.

De Leonardis, O. (1988a) 'I diritti difficili', *Democrazia e diritto*, 2/3, 71–96.

De Leonardis, O. (1988b) 'Il ciclo di una politica: la riforma psichiatrica', in C. Donolo, F. Fichera, *Le vie dell'innovazione*, Feltrinelli, Milan.

De Leonardis, O. (1988c) 'L'emergenza quotidiana e i dilemmi del magistrato: il problema psichiatrico nel lavoro della pretura penale', in O. De Leonardis, G. Gallio, D. Mauri, T. Pitch (eds), *Curare e punire*, Unicopli, Milan.

De Leonardis, O. (1990) *Il terzo escluso*, Feltrinelli, Milan.

De Nardis, P. (1988) *L'equivoco sistema*, Franco Angeli, Milan.

De Stroebel, G. (1985) 'Analisi critica della statistica giudiziaria e criminale in tema di giustizia minorile dal 1947 ad oggi', in L. Bergonzini, M. Pavarini (1985) (eds), *Potere giudiziario, enti locali e giustizia minorile*, Il Mulino, Bologna.

Debuyst, C. (1981) (ed.), *Dangerosite et justice*, Medicine et Higiene, Geneva.

Dell'Acqua, G., Mezzina, R. (1988) (eds), *Il folle gesto. Perizia psichiatrica, manicomio giudiziario, carcere nella pratica dei servizi di salute mentale a Trieste (1987–1988)*, Sapere 2000, Rome.

Di Lazzaro, A. (1988) 'Le misure alternative alla detenzione prima e dopo la legge Gozzini', *Inchiesta*, XVIII, 79/80, 27–40.

Diotima (1987) (ed.), *Il pensiero della differenza sessuale*, La Tartaruga, Milan.

Dominijanni, I. (1988) 'Sguardi diversi sullo stupro', *Il Manifesto*, 12 April.

Dominijanni, I. (1989) 'Donne si nasce, differenti si diventa. L'eguaglianza e il percorso femminista', *il Bimestrale*, 1, 74–78.

Donolo, C., Fichera, F. (1988) *Le vie dell'innovazione*, Feltrinelli, Milan.

Dosi, G. (1985) 'Azione imputabile e responsabilità minorile', *Esperienze di giustizia minorile*, XXXII, 1, 37–90.

Douglas, M. (1986) *How Institutions Think*, University of Syracuse Press, Syracuse.

Douglas, M., Wildavsky, AA. (1983) *Risk and Culture*, University of California Press, Berkeley.

Dowd Hall, J. (1983) 'The Mind That Burns in Each Body': Women, Rape and Racial Violence', in A. Snitow, Christine Stansell, Sharon Thompson (eds), *Powers of Desire. The Politics of Sexuality*, Monthly Review Press, New York.

Dresser, R. (1982) 'Ulysses and the Psychiatrists: a Legal and Policy Analysis of the

Voluntary Commitment Contract', *Harvard Civil Rights Civil Liberties Law Review*.

Durkheim, E. (1963) *Le regole del metodo sociologico*, Milan, Comunità.

Dusi, P. (1982) 'Categorie giuridiche e categorie socio-psicologiche', in M.P. Cuomo, G. La Greca, L. Viggiani, *Giudici, psicologi e delinquenza giovanile*, Giuffré, Milan.

Dworkin, A. (1982) *Pornography. Men Possessing Women*, The Women's Press, London.

Elster, J. (1978) *Logic and Society*, Wiley, New York.

Elster, J. (1983) *Ulisse e le sirene*, Il Mulino, Bologna.

Empey, L.T. (1978) *American Delinquency. Its Meaning and Construction*, Ill, Dorsey, Homewood.

Empey, L.T. (1979) (ed.), *The Future of Childhood and Juvenile Justice*, University of Virginia Press, Charlottesville.

Erikson, K.T. (1961) 'Notes on the Sociology of Deviance', *Social Problems*, IX, 2, 307–314.

Faccioli, F. (1984) 'Il sociologo e la criminalità. Riflessioni sulle origini della criminologia critica in Italia', *Dei delitti e delle pene*, I, 1, 602–642.

Faccioli, F. (1987) 'Il "comando" difficile. Considerazioni su donne e controllo nel carcere femminile', in T. Pitch (ed.) *Diritto e rovescio*, ESI, Naples.

Faccioli, F. (1988) 'Aspetti della giustizia penale', in ISTAT e AIS (ed.), *Immagini della società italiana*, Istat, Rome.

Faccioli, F. (1988a) 'Devianza e controllo istituzionale', in Consiglio Nazionale dei Minori, *I minori in Italia* (edited by G. Statera), Franco Angeli, Milan.

Faccioli, F. (1988b) 'I percorsi della sociologia: teorie sociologiche e modelli di controllo', in F. Faccioli, T. Pitch (eds), *Senza patente. Una ricerca sull'intervento penale sulle minorenni a Roma*, Franco Angeli, Milan.

Faccioli, F. and Pitch, T. (1988) *Senza patente. Una ricerca sull'intervento penale sulle minorenni a Roma*, Franco Angeli, Milan.

Fadiga, L., Gerratana, G., Occulto, R. (1985) 'L'evoluzione della delinquenza giovanile nell'ultimo decennio', *Esperienze di giustizia minorile*, XXXII, 1, 7–31.

Febbrajo, A. (1975) *Funzionalismo strutturale e sociologia del diritto in Luhmann*, Giuffré, Milan.

Feltsiner, W.L.F., Abel, R.L., Sarat, A. (1980–81) 'The Emergence and Transformation of Disputes', *Law and Society* 15, 3–4, 631–654.

Ferracuti, F. (1986) 'Intervento' al *V seminario nazionale per professori italiani di discipline criminologiche*, Siracusa, 9–11 October.

Ferrajoli, L. (1977) 'Ordine pubblico e legislazione eccezionale', *La questione criminale*, III, 3, 361–404.

Ferrajoli, L. (1984) 'Emergenza penale e crisi della giurisdizione', *Dei delitti e delle pene*, II, 2, 271–293.

Ferrajoli, L. (1985) 'Il diritto penale minimo', *Dei delitti e delle pene*, III, 3, 493–524.

Ferrajoli, L., Zolo, D. (1977) 'Marxismo e questione criminale', *La questione criminale*, III, 1, 97–132.

Ferrajoli, L., Zolo, D. (1978) *Democrazia autoritaria e capitalismo maturo*, Feltrinelli, Milan.

Ferrarese, M.R. (1984) *L'istituzione difficile. La magistratura tra professione e sistema politico*, ESI, Naples.

Ferrari, V. (1980) 'L'analisi funzionale in sociologia del dirrito', *Sociologia del diritto*, VII, 1, 43–70.

Ferrari, V. (1987) *Le funzioni del diritto*, Laterza, Bari.

Fiandaca, G. (1984) 'La tipizzazione del pericolo', *Dei delitti e delle pene*, II, 3, 441–472.

Fiandaca, G. (1987) 'I presupposti della responsabilità penale tra dogmatica e scienze sociali', *Dei delitti e delle pene*, V, 2, 243–268.

Fine, B. (1987) 'What is Social About Social Control', *Contemporary Crises*, 10, 3, 321–327.

Flax, J. (1987) 'Postmodernism and Gender. Relations in Feminist Theory', *Signs*, XII, 41, 621–643.

Flax, J. (1988) 'Are Postmodernist Feminist Theories of Justice Possible?', relazione presentata al seminario *Equality and Difference: Gender Dimensions in Political Thought, Justice, and Morality*, Istituto Universitario Europeo, Florence, 1–3 December.

Forato, G. (1982) 'La ricerca della verità nella pratica giuridica e psicologica', in M.P. Cuomo, G. La Greca, L. Viggiani (eds), *Giudici, psicologi e delinquenza giovanile*, Giuffré, Milan.

Fornari, U. (1986) 'Problemi clinici in psichiatria forense', relazione presentata al *V seminario nazionale per professori italiani di discipline criminologiche*, Siracusa, 9–11 October.

Foucault, M. (1976) *Sorvegliare e punire*, Einaudi, Turin.

Foucault, M. (1976a) *Io... Pierre Riviére*, Einaudi, Turin.

Foucault, M. (1976b) *Histoire de la sexualité. La volonté de savoir*, Gallimard, Paris.

Fox Keller, E. (1987) *Sul genere e la scienza*, Garzanti, Milan.

Franchini, A., Introna, F. (1972) *Delinquenza minorile*, Cleup, Padova.

Friedman, L.M. (1975) *Il sistema giuridico nella prospettiva delle scienze sociali*, Il Mulino, Bologna.

Gallio, G. (1988) 'Eclisse della pericolosità e istanze di controllo nell'intervento psichiatrico: i servizi alla prova di nuove strategie e culture della responsabilità', in O. De Leonardis, G. Gallio, D. Mauri, T. Pitch (eds), *Curare e punire*, Unicopli, Milan.

Galzigna, M. (1984) 'Gli infortuni della libertà', introduzione a E.J. Georget, *Il crimine e la colpa*, Marsilio, Venice.

Gandus, N. (1988) 'I "casi di pretura" tra intervento terapeutico e intervento penale', in O. De Leonardis, G. Gallio, D. Mauri, T. Pitch (eds), *Curare e punire*, Unicopli, Milan.

Gandus, et al. (1990) *Riforma dei reati di violenza sessuale e nuovo codice di procedura penale*, Circolo della Rosa, Rome.

Garland, D. (1985) *Punishment and Welfare: A History of Penal Strategies*, Aldershot, Brodfield.

Gatti, U. (1988) 'L'accertamento dell'imputabilità e della pericolosità sociale alla luce della situazione esistente in alcuni paesi europei', in O. De Leonardis, G. Gallio, D. Mauri, T. Pitch (eds), *Curare e punire*, Unicopli, Milan.

Gatti, U., Bandini, T. (1970) 'Istituti di rieducazione e identità negativa', *Rassegna di criminologia*, I, 1, 10–32.

Geertz, C. (1988) *Antropologia interpretativa*, Il Mulino, Bologna.

Georget, E.J. (1984) *Il crimine e la colpa*, Marsilio, Venice.

Giannichedda, M.G. (1986) 'Salute, diritti, controllo sociale. Modelli di psichiatria dopo la riforma', *Dei delitti e delle pene*, IV, 1, 5–26.

Giannichedda, M.G. (1987) 'Schede e documento del Coordinamento nazionale associazioni di familiari e cittadini per la riforma psichiatrica', in M.G. Ginni-chedda, F. Ongaro Basaglia (eds), *Psichiatria, tossicodipendenze, perizia*, Franco Angeli, Milan.

Giasanti, A. (1985) 'Marginalità giovanile e società complessa', in G. Ponti (eds), *Giovani responsabilità e giustizia*, Giuffré, Milan.

Gibson, M. (1987) 'Marginalità convergenti. L'immagine borghese della prostituta, 1850–1915', in T. Pitch (eds), *Diritto e rovescio*, ESI, Naples.

Giddens, A. (1979) *Nuove regole del metodo sociologico*, Il Mulino, Bologna.

Giddens, A. (1987) *Social Theory and Modern Sociology*, Stanford University Press, Stanford.

Giglioli, P., Dal Lago, A. (eds) (1983) *Etnometodologia*, Il Mulino, Bologna.

Gilligan, C. (1987) *Con voce di donna*, Feltrinelli, Milan.

Goffman, E. (1963) *Stigma. Notes on the Management of Spoiled Identity*, Prentice Hall, Englewall Cliffs.

Goffman, E. (1968) *Asylums*, Einaudi, Turin.

Greenberg, D. (ed.) (1977) *Corrections and Punishment*, Sage, Beverly Hills.

Greenberg, D. (ed.) (1981) *Crime and Capitalism*, Mayfield Publishing Company, Palo Alto.

Greenberg, D., Humphries, D. (1981) 'The Cooptation of Fixed Sentencing Reform', in D. Greenberg (eds) *Crime and Capitalism*, Mayfield, Palo Alto.

Groppi, A. (1983–4) 'Un pezzo di mercanzia di cui il mercante fa quel che ne vuole', *Annali della Fondazione Lelio e Lisli Basso*, VII, Franco Angeli, Milan.

Gusfield, J.R. (1966) *Symbolic Crusade, Status Politics and the American Temperance Movement*, University of Illinois Press, Urbana.

Gusfield, J.R. (1975) 'Categories of Ownership and Responsibility in Social Issues', *Journal of Drug Issues*, 7–15.

Gusfield, J.R. (1981) *The Culture of Public Problems. Drinking Driving and the Symbolic Order*, University of Chicago Press, Chicago.

Hall, S. *et al.* (1978) *Policing the Crisis*, Macmillan, London.

Hanmer, J., Saunders, S. (1984) *Well Founded Fear*, Hutchinson, London.

Harding, T.W. (1980) 'Du danger, de la dangerosité et de l'usage medical de termes affectivement charges', *Deviance et Société*, 4.

Heidensohn, F. (1986) 'Models of Justice: Portia or Persephone?', *The International Journal of the Sociology of Law*, n. 3–4.

Henderson, L.N. (1985) 'The Wrongs of Victim's Rights', *Stanford Law Review*, April, 937–1021.

Hirschman, A.D. (1982) *Lealtà, defezione, protesta*, Bompiani, Milan.

Hirschmann, N.J. (1992) *Rethinking Obligation. A Feminist Method for Political Theory*, Ithaca, Cornell University Press.

Howe, A. (1987) '"Social Injury" Revisited: Towards a Feminist Theory of Social Justice', *The International Journal of the Sociology of Law*, XV, 4, 423–438.

Hulsman, L. (1982) *Peines Perdues*, Le Centurion, Paris.

Hulsman, L. (1983) 'Abolire il sistema penale?' (Intervista a...), *Dei delitti e delle pene*, I, 1, 71–89.

Irigaray, L. (1985) *Etica della differenza sessuale*, Feltrinelli, Milan.

Irigaray, L. (1988) 'Il sapere e le origini', *Fluttuaria*, 5, 13–16.

Janowitz, M. (1975) 'Sociological Theory and Social Control', *The American Journal of Sociology*, 81, 1, 82–108.

Jonas, A. (1984) *The Imperative of Responsibility*, The University of California Press, Chicago–London.

King, M., Piper, C. (1990) *How the Law Thinks About Children*, Gower, Aldershot.

Kitsuse, J.I. (1962) 'Societal Reactions to Behavior: Problems of Theory and Method', *Social Problems*, IX, 3, 247–265.

Klein, D. (1988) 'Women Offenders, Victims and False Labels', paper presented at the *X International Congress on Criminology*, Hamburg.

Krisberg, B., Austin, J. (1978) 'The Children of Ishmael, Mayfield Publishing Company, California.

Lagostena Bassi, T. (1979) 'Il diritto delle donne di proporre una legge', *Rinascita*, 46.

Lasch, C. (1984) *The Minimal Self. Psychic Survival in Troubled Times*, W.W. Norton, New York.

Lea, J., Young, J. (1984) *What Is to Be Done About Law and Order?*, Penguin, Harmondsworth.

Lemert, E.M. (1951) *Social Pathology*, Hill Book Company, New York–Toronto–London.

Lemert, E.M. (1981) *Devianza, problemi sociali e forme di controllo*, Giuffré, Milan.

Libreria delle donne di Milano (1983) 'Più donne che uomini', *Sottosopra*, January.

Libreria delle donne di Milano (1987) *Non credere di avere dei diritti*, Rosenberg e Sellier, Turin.

Libreria delle donne di Milano (1988) 'Lettera', *Il foglio del Paese delle donne*, I, 20–21–22–23 September.

Libreria delle donne di Milano (1990).

Luberto, S., De Fazio, F. (1986) 'La prassi della perizia psichiatrica', relazione al *V seminario nazionale per professori italiani di discipline criminologiche*, Siracusa, 9–11 October.

Luhmann, N. (1977) *Sociologia del diritto*, Laterza, Bari.

Luhmann, N. (1978) *Stato di diritto e sistema sociale*, Guida, Naples.

Luker, K. (1984) *Abortion and the Politics of Motherhood*, University of California Press, Berkeley.

Manacorda, A. (1982) *Il Manicomio Giudiziario. Teoria e prassi di una istituzione*, De Donato, Bari.

Manacorda, A. (1988) (ed.) *Folli e reclusi*, La Casa Usher, Florence.

Mancina, C. (1988) 'Un conflitto dentro e oltre la storia', in M. L. Boccia, I. Peretti (eds) *Il genere della rappresentanza*, Editori Riuniti, Rome.

Marconi, P. (1979) *La libertà selvaggia*, Marsilio, Venice.

Marconi, P. (1983) 'La percettibilità del disordine e il bisogno di sicurezza', *Dei delitti e delle pene*, I, 2, 269–282.

Marconi, P. (1983a) 'La strategia abolizionista di Louk Hulsman', *Dei delitti e delle pene*, I, 1, 221–238.

Marconi, P. (1984) *Economie della giustizia penale*, Marsilio, Pardova.

Marinelli, A. (1988) *Struttura dell'ordine e funzione del diritto*, Franco Angeli, Milan.

Marsh, J.C., Geist, A., Caplan, N. (1982) *Rape and the Limits of Law Reform*, Auburn Publishing House, Boston.

Matthews, R., Young, J. (eds) (1986) *Confronting Crime*, Sage, London.

Mathiesen, T. (1974) *The Politics of Abolition. Essay in Political Action Theory*, Universitetsforlaget, Oslo.

Mathiesen, T. (1983) 'The Future of Control Systems. The Case of Norway', in D. Garland, P. Young (eds), *The Power to Punish*, Heinemann, London.

Matza, D. (1976) *Come si diventa devianti*, Il Mulino, Bologna.
Mauri, D. (1983) (ed.), *La libertà è terapeutica?*, Feltrinelli, Milan.
Mauri, D. (1988) 'I rapporti tra psichiatria e giustizia penale negli Stati Uniti', in O. De Leonardis, G. Gallio, D. Mauri, T. Pitch (ed.), *Curare e punire*, Unicopli, Milan.
Mauri, D., Pitch, T. (1990) 'Diritto alla saluete e disturbo psichico nel carcere di S. Vittore', in IReR (editor), *Tensioni e nuovi bisogni nella città in transformazione*, Franco Angeli, Milan.
Mazzei, D. (1984) 'Sulla capacità di intendere e di volere in età evolutiva', *Esperienze di Rieducazione*, XXXI, 2, 7–37.
McKinnon, C. (1979) *Sexual Harassment of Working Women: A Case of Sex Discrimination*, Yale University Press, New Haven.
McKinnon, C. (1987) *Feminism Unmodified. Discourses on Life and Law*, Harvard University Press, Cambridge.
McNickle, R.V. (1977) 'Rape as a Social Problem: A Byproduct of the Feminist Movement', *Social Problems*, 1, 75–89.
Mead, G.H. (1966) *Mente, sé e società*, G. Barbera, Florence.
Melossi, D. (1980) 'Oltre il Panopticon. Per uno studio delle strategie di controllo sociale nel capitalismo del ventesimo secolo', *La questione criminale*, VI, 2/3, 277–361.
Melossi, D. (1983) 'A Politics Without a State: the Concepts of "State" and "Social Control" from European to American Social Science', 205–222, in S. Spitzer (ed.), *Research in Law, Deviance and Social Control*, 5, JAI Press, Greenwich.
Melossi, D., Pavarini, M. (1976) *Carcere e fabbrica*, Il Mulino, Bologna.
Melucci, A. (1985) 'The Symbolic Challenge of Contemporary Movements', *Social Research*, LII, 4, 789–816.
Melucci, A. (1987) *La libertà che cambia*, Unicopli, Milan.
Merlin, L., Barberis, C. (1955) (ed.), *Lettere dalle case chiuse*, Edizioni Avanti, Milan–Rome.
Merry, S.E. (1981) *Urban Danger. Life in a Neighborhood of Strangers*, Temple University Press, Philadelphia.
Merton, R.K. (1971) *Teoria e struttura sociale*, Il Mulino, Bologna.
Micheli, G.A., Carabelli, G. (1986) *Sofferenza psichica in scenari urbani*, Unicopli, Milan.
Micheli, G.A. (1986) 'La dimensione sociologica dei servizi psichiatrici', in P.P. Donati (ed.), *Salute e complessità sociale*, Franco Angeli, Milan.
Miers, D.R. (1983) 'Compensation and Conceptions of Victims of Crime', *Victimology*, VIII, 1/2, 204–212.
Minow, M. (1990) *Making All the Difference*, Cornell University Press, Ithaca.
Morgan, P. (1981) 'From Battered Wife to Program Client', *Kapitalistate*, 9, 17–40.
Mosconi, G. (1986) 'Riferimenti per un'alternativa reale al carcere', *Dei delitti e delle pene*, IV, 2, 277–315.
Mosconi, G. (1986) 'La legge Gozzini, una riforma nel conflitto', *Critica del diritto*, n. 40–41.
Mosconi, G. (1988) 'Le trasformazioni della pena nello spazio della cultura diffusa', *Inchiesta*, XVIII, 79/80, 1–12.
NDC (National Deviancy Conference) (ed.) (1980) *Permissiveness and Social Control. The Fate of the 60s Legislation*, Macmillan, London.
NDC/CSE (Conference of Socialist Economists) (ed.) (1979) *Capitalism and the Rule of Law. From Deviancy Theory to Marxism*, Macmillan, London.

Nelken, D. (1985) 'Community Involvement in Crime Control: if Community is the Answer, What is the Question?' relazione presentata al convegno *Social Control and Justice: Inside and/or Outside the Law*, Gerusalemme, 28 March–3 April.

Novello, M. (1987) 'Malattia e responsabilità', in M.G. Giannichedda, F. Ongaro Basaglia (eds), *Psichiatria, tossicodipendenze, perizia*, Franco Angeli, Milan.

Okin Moller, S. (1989) *Justice, Gender and the Family*, Basic Books, New York.

Olgiati, V., Astori, M. (1988) 'Difesa privata armata in Italia: dalla supplenza all'appalto del controllo sociale diffuso', relazione presentata al *Congresso mondiale dell'Associazione Internazionale di Sociologia del Diritto*, Bologna, 30 May–3 June.

Parsons, T. (1962) 'The Law and Social Control', in W. Evan (ed.), *Law and Sociology*, The Free Press of Glencoe, New York.

Parsons, T. (1965) *Il sistema sociale*, Comunità, Milan.

Parton, N. (1981) 'Child Abuse, Social Anxiety and Welfare', *The British Journal of Sociology*, 11, 391–414.

Pateman, C. (1988) *The Sexual Contract*, Stanford University Press, Stanford.

Pavarini, M. (1975) 'Il socialmente pericoloso nell'attività di prevenzione', *Rivista italiana di diritto e procedura penale*, XVIII, 2.

Pavarini, M. (1981) *Introduzione a... la criminologia*, Le Monnier, Florence.

Pavarini, M. (1983) 'La crisi della prevenzione speciale tra istanze garantiste e ideologie neoliberiste', in G. Cotturri, M. Ramat (eds), *Quali garanzie*, De Donato, Bari.

Pavarini, M. (1985) 'Il sistema della giustizia penale tra riduzionismo e abolizionismo', *Dei delitti e delle pene*, III, 3, 525–553.

Pavarini, M. (1986) 'Fuori delle mura del carcere: la dislocazione dell'ossessione correzionale', *Dei delitti e delle pene*, IV, 2, 251–276.

Pavarini, M. (1987) 'Riflessioni in merito alle modifiche sull'ordinamento penitenziario', *Marginalità e Società*, n. 1–2.

Pavarini, M. (1988) 'Misure alternative al carcere e decarcerizzazione: un rapporto problematico', *Inchiesta*, XVIII, 79/80, 49–53.

Pfohl, S. (1978) *Predicting Dangerousness. The Social Construction of Psychiatric Reality*, D.C. Heat and Company, Lexington.

Pfohl, S. (1977) 'The Discovery of Child Abuse', *Social Problems*, XXIV, 3, 310–323.

Pitch, T. (1982) *La devianza*, La Nuova Italia, Florence.

Pitch, T. (1983) 'Sociology of Law in Italy', *Journal of Law and Society*, X, 1, 119–134.

Pitch, T. (1983a) 'Tra diritti sociali e cittadinanza. Il movimento delle donne e la legge sulla violenza sessuale', *Problemi del Socialismo*, 27/28, 192–214.

Pitch, T. (1984) 'La nuova legge sulla violenza sessuale', *Dei delitti e delle pene*, II, 2, 317–323.

Pitch, T. (1985) 'Critical Criminology, the Construction of Social Problems and the Question of Rape', *The International Journal of the Sociology of Law*, 13, 35–46.

Pitch, T. (1986) 'Viaggio intorno alla "criminologia". Discutendo con i realisti', *Dei delitti e delle pene*, IV, 3, 469–488.

Pitch, T. (1987) (ed.) *Diritto e rovescio. Studi sulle donne e il controllo sociale*, ESI, Naples.

Pitch, T. (1988) 'Che cos'è il controllo sociale', 21–44, in O. De Leonardis, G. Gallio, D. Mauri, T. Pitch (eds), *Curare e punire*, Unicopli, Milan.

Pitch, T. (1992) 'Quale giustizia per le donne. Appunti per un dibattito', in E. Campelli *et al.*, *Donne in carcere*, Feltrinelli, Milan.

Piven Fox, F., Cloward, R. (1972) *Regulating the Poor*, Vintage Books, New York.

Pizzorno, A. (1986) Intervento al seminario *Pericolosità sociale, psichiatria, controllo sociale*, Dipartimento di Sociologia, Falcoltà di Scienze Politiche, Università di Milan, 19–20 April.

Platt, A. (1973) 'Prospects for a Radical Criminology in the United States', relazione al *I Convegno del Gruppo Europeo per lo Studio della Devianza e del Controllo Sociale*, Impruneta, 13–16 September.

Platt, A. (1975) *L'invenzione della delinquenza*, Guaraldi, Florence.

Platt, A., Takagi, P. (1978) 'Intellettuali per la legge e l'ordine: una critica dei nuovi "realisti"', *La questione criminale*, IV, 2, 217–251.

Platt, A., Takagi, P. (1981) (eds) *Crime and Social Justice*, Macmillan, London.

Ponti, G. (1985) (ed.) *Giovani responsabilità e giustizia*, Giuffré, Milan.

Ponti, G.L. (1985a) *Guida alla perizia psichiatrica*, Scuola di specializzazione in Criminologia clinica, Università di Milano.

Pulitanò, D. (1988) 'L'imputabilità come problema giuridico', in O. De Leonardis, G. Gallio, D. Mauri, T. Pitch (eds), *Curare e punire*, Unicopli, Milan.

Rabine, L.W. (1988) 'A Feminist Politics of Non-Identity', *Feminist Studies*, XIV, 1, 11–31.

Rafter, N.H. (1985) *Partial Justice. Women in State Prisons 1800–1935*, Northeastern University Press, Boston.

Reamer, F.G. (1982) *Ethical Dilemmas in Social Service*, University of Columbia Press, New York.

Reinarman, C. (1988) 'The Social Construction of an Alcohol Problem', *Theory and Society*, 17, 91–120.

Resta, E. (1983) 'Il diritto penale premiale. "Nuove" strategie di controllo sociale, *Dei delitti e delle pene*, I, 1, 41–70.

Resta, E. (1985) 'La dismisura dei sistemi penali', *Dei delitti e delle pene*, III, 3, 475–492.

Ricoeur, P. (1986) *La semantica dell'azione*, Jaca Book, Milan.

Robert, P. (1982) 'La crise de la notion de dangerosité', *Rassegna di criminologia*, 2.

Ross, E.A. (1922) *Social Control*, Macmillan, New York.

Rubin, G. (1981) 'The Leather Menace: Comments on Politics and S/M', in *Coming to Power*, Samois, Berkeley.

Rusche, G., Kirchheimer, O. (1978) *Pena e struttura sociale*, Il Mulino, Bologna.

Santarsiero, G. (1985) 'L'imputabilità tra scienza e prassi', *Esperienze di giustizia minorile*, XXXII, 1, 124–137.

Saraceno, C. (1987) *Pluralità e mutamento*, Franco Angeli, Milan.

Saraceno, C. (1988) 'La struttura di genere della cittadinanza', *Democrazia e diritto*, XXVIII, 1, 273–295.

Scheerer, S. (1983) 'L'abolizionismo nella criminologia contemporanea', *Dei delitti e delle pene*, I, 3, 525–540.

Schlossman, S.L. (1977) *Love and the American Delinquent*, University of Chicago Press, Chicago.

Schwendinger, H., Schwendinger, J.R. (1973) 'A Report to the European Group at the Florence Conference', relazione al I Convegno del Gruppo Europeo per lo studio della Devianza e del Controllo Sociale, Impruneta, 13–16 September.

Schwendinger, H., Schwendinger, J.R. (1983) *Rape and Inequality*, Sage, London.

Scott, J.W. (1988) 'Deconstructing Equality-Versus-Difference: Or, The Uses of Poststructuralist Theory for Feminism', *Feminist Studies*, XIV, 1, 33–50.

Scraton, P., South, N. (1984) 'The Ideological Construction of the Hidden Economy: Private Justice and Work Related Crime', *Contemporary Crises*, 8, 1, 1–19.

Scull, A. (1977) *Decarceration*, Prentice Hall, New Jersey.

Scull, A. (1982) 'Community Corrections: Panacea, Progress or Pretence', in R. Abel (ed.), *The Politics of Informal Justice*, Academic Press, New York.

Sen, A. (1985) *Commodities and Capabilities*, Amsterdam, North Holland.

Senzani, G. (1970) *L'esclusione anticipata*, Jaca Book, Milan.

Sergio, G. (1982) 'Sistema penale e devianza minorile', in M.P. Cuomo, G. La Greca, L. Viggiani (eds), *Giudici, psicologi e delinquenza giovanile*, Giuffré, Milan.

Sezione Femminile Del, PCI (1986) (eds) *Dalle donne la forza delle donne. Carta itinerante*.

Shearing, C.D., Stenning, P.C. (1985) 'From the Panopticon to Disney World: The Development of Discipline', in A.N. Dobb, E.L. Greenspan (eds), *Perspectives in Criminal Law*, Canada Law Book, Ontario.

Silbernagl, M. (1987) 'Il diritto penale senza colpevolezza? Appunti critici sul processo di dissoluzione della categoria della colpevolezza nel diritto penale preventivo orientato alle conseguenze', *Dei delitti e delle pene*, V, 2, 269–313.

Snider, L. 'Legal Reform and Social Control: the Dangers of Abolishing Rape', *The International Journal of the Sociology of Law*, XIII, 4, 337–356.

Snitow, A., Stansell, C. Thompson, S. (1983) (eds) *Powers of Desire. The Politics of Sexuality*, The Monthly Review Press, New York.

Spagnoletti, M.T. (1985) 'Il minore non imputabile', *Esperienze di giustizia minorile*, XXXII, 1, 68–79.

Spector, M. (1981) 'Oltre il crimine: come controllare chi disturba la pace sociale', *La questione criminale*, VII, 2, 183–217.

Stanworth, M. (ed.) (1987) *Reproductive Technologies*, University of Minnesota Press, Minneapolis.

Stark, E., Flitcraft, A., Frazier, W. (1979) 'Medicine and Patriarchal Violence: The Social Construction of a Private Event', *International Journal of Health Services*, IX, 3, 461–493.

Sutherland, E. (1945) 'Is "White Collar Crime" Crime?', *American Sociological Review*, 10, 132–139.

Tappan, P. (1947) 'Who Is the Criminal?', *American Sociological Review*, 12, 96–102.

Taylor, I., Walton, P., Young, J. (1975) *Criminologia sotto accusa*, Guaraldi, Florence.

Teodori, M.A. (1986) (ed.) *Lucciole in lotta. La prostituzione come lavoro*, Sapere 2000, Rome.

Teubner (1983) 'Substantive and Reflexive Elements in Modern Law', *Law and Society Review*, 17.

Tomeo, V. (1981) *Il diritto come struttura del conflitto*, Franco Angeli, Milan.

Touraine, A. (1985) 'An Introduction to the Study of Social Movements', *Social Research*, LII, 4, 749–787.

Traverso, G.B. (1979) 'The dangerous offender legislation. A critical understanding', *Rassegna di criminologia*, X, 2, 377–398.

Treves, R. (1972) *Giustizia e giudici nella società italiana*, Laterza, Bari.

Treves, R. (1987) *Introduzione alla sociologia del diritto*, Einaudi, Turin.

Turnaturi, G. (1991) *Associati per amore*, Feltrinelli, Milan.

Turnaturi, G., Donolo, C. (1988) 'Familismi morali', in C. Donolo, F. Fichera, *Le vie dell'innovazione*, Feltrinelli, Milan.

Vaccaro, A. (1982) 'Il perdono giudiziale', in AA.VV., *Risposte giudiziarie alla criminalità minorile*, Unicopli, Milan.

Vaccaro, A. (1982a) 'L'accertamento della maturità in astratto e in concreto nell'ambito della risposta penale alla devianza minorile', in M.P. Cuomo, G. La Greca, L. Viggiani (eds), *Giudici, psicologi e delinquenza giovanile*, Giuffré, Milan.

Van Den Haag, E. (1975) *Punishing Criminals*, Basic Books, New York.

Veca, S. (1982) *La società giusta*, Il Saggiatore, Milan.

Vega, J. (1988) 'Coercion and Consent: Classical Liberal Concepts in Texts on Sexual Violence', *International Journal of the Sociology of Law*, XVI, 1, 75–89.

Ventimiglia, C. (1987) *La differenza negata*, Franco Angeli, Milan.

Vercellone, P. (1982) 'L'imputabilità e punibilità dei minorenni nella legge penale italiana', in M.P. Cuomo, G. La Greca, L. Viggiani (eds), *Giudici psicologi e delinquenza giovanile*, Giuffré, Milan.

Viano, E. 'Victim's Rights and the Constitution: Reflections in a Bicentennial', *Crime and Delinquency*, XXXIII, 4, 438–451.

Virgilio, M. (1987) 'La donna nel Codice Rocco', in T. Pitch (ed.), *Diritto e rovescio*, ESI, Naples.

von Hirsch, A. (1976) *Doing Justice. The Choice of Punishments*, Basic Books, New York.

Walkowitz, J. (1987) 'Vizi maschili e virtù femministe. Il femminismo e la politica nei confronti della prostituzione nella Gran Bretagna del XIX secolo', in T. Pitch (ed.), *Diritto e rovescio*, ESI, Naples.

Walzer, M. (1983) *Sfere di giustizia*, Feltrinelli, Milan.

Walzer, M. (1985) *Esodo e rivoluzione*, Feltrinelli, Milan.

White, M. (1956) *La rivolta contro il formalismo*, Il Mulino, Bologna.

Wilson, J.Q. (1975) *Thinking About Crime*, Basic Books, New York.

Wilson, J.Q., Herrnstein, R.J. (1985) *Crime and Human Nature*, Simon and Schuster, New York.

Wolgast, E. (1991) *La grammatica della giustizia*, Editori Riuniti, Rome.

Young, J. (1986) 'Il fallimento della criminologia: per un realismo radicale', *Dei delitti e delle pene*, IV, 3, 387–415.

Name index

Subject index